HEALTHSPANGEVITY™

Unlocking Longevity and Vitality

Live Longer, Live Well

Your Practical Guide to Optimal Health

Dr. Catherine Oseni, Pharm.D., FAAMFM, ABAAHP, FICT

Dr. Olusegun Oseni, M.D., FCCP, DABSM

ISBN: 9798284946862

DEDICATION

This book is dedicated, first and foremost, to God—the ultimate healer—for the priceless gift of health, the miracle of healing, and the privilege of guiding others on their wellness journeys.

To our three incredible sons—David, Jonathan, and Joshua—your love is our compass, your spirit our fuel. Your unwavering support ignites our passion and gives purpose to our mission.

To our parents, family, and extended community—our church family, pastors, mentors, colleagues, friends, and the many lives we've had the honor to touch—your wisdom, encouragement, and boundless love have shaped this vision in ways words cannot capture.

To the exceptional teams at Alpha Care Wellness Center, Lung and Sleep Specialists of North Texas, and our wonderful colleagues and staff at The Center for Cancer and Blood Disorders, Texas—your dedication and compassion inspire us daily.

To our patients and clients, thank you for entrusting us with your health. And to the relentless health warriors who refuse to accept aging as a slow descent, proof that growing older is not about growing weaker, but about cultivating vitality, resilience, and unstoppable energy at every stage of life.

To the seekers of truth, the bold trailblazers who challenge the status quo—you recognize that true wellness isn't found in prescriptions but in prevention. You understand that while conventional medicine often stops managing symptoms, real transformation begins when we nurture the body, mind, and spirit from within.

This book is for those ready to defy expectations and unlock the secrets to youthful aging, longevity, and optimal well-being. Within these pages, you'll discover science-backed strategies and natural, empowering methods to help your body heal, regenerate, and thrive. From cutting-edge healing therapies to lifestyle practices that slow aging and amplify performance, this is your roadmap to a vibrant life.

Aging is inevitable. Decline is optional. Together, let's rewrite the rules—becoming the strongest, healthiest, and most radiant versions of ourselves.

The journey begins now.

DISCLAIMER

This book is designed to inspire and inform, not to diagnose, treat, or replace professional medical advice. Think of it as a guide to unlocking longevity and vitality—filled with science-backed insights and practical strategies to support your health journey. However, it's not a substitute for personalized care from your healthcare provider.

Always consult with a qualified medical professional before making any significant changes to your diet, exercise, or wellness routines. Your health is unique, and professional guidance ensures that your path to longevity is safe and effective.

Curious about the science behind these strategies? For a comprehensive list of studies and research supporting the information in this book, simply scan this QR code:

FOREWORD

We are living in an era where millions suffer and die from diseases that are, in many cases, entirely preventable. Heart attacks, strokes, cancer, dementia—the list goes on. And while conventional medicine continues to chase symptoms, it has largely failed to address the root causes of these chronic conditions. That's why it brings me such immense hope and joy to introduce a book that doesn't just patch the problem—it rewrites the entire health paradigm.

It is my true honor to write the foreword for *Unlocking Longevity, Healthspangevity™, and Vitality*—a groundbreaking and timely contribution to the field of integrative medicine by my esteemed colleague and friend, Dr. Olusegun Oseni, and his brilliant partner in life and purpose, Catherine Oseni.

As a cardiologist who has spent decades championing the foundations of true health: real food, quality sleep, movement, sunlight, meaningful connection, and love, I can say with certainty that this book is a masterclass in healing. But more than that, it's a blueprint for *thriving*. The Osenis introduce us to the concept of *Healthspangevity™*, the beautiful synergy of healthspan and longevity. Not just living longer—but living *better*.

Dr. Olusegun Oseni is a rare and remarkable physician. Board-certified in internal medicine, pulmonary care, critical care, and sleep medicine, his medical knowledge runs deep. Yet what truly sets him apart is his unwavering focus on *root-cause resolution*. He's not content with disease management—he's committed to helping the body do what it was designed to do: *heal*. By blending advanced science with time-honored, holistic practices, Dr. Oseni is forging a new path for what medicine should be—proactive, personalized, and profoundly transformational.

Dr. Catherine Oseni is a force of healing in her own right. With a strong foundation in clinical pharmacy and nearly two decades of experience in functional and metabolic medicine, she brings both heart and science to every interaction. Her superpower is translating complex biochemistry into simple, personalized protocols that help people regain energy, rebalance hormones, and reclaim joy. Her work has changed thousands of lives—and this book will undoubtedly change countless more.

Together, the Osenis are a powerhouse. And what they've created here is nothing short of a gift to the world.

Unlocking Longevity, Healthspangevity™, and Vitality is both inspiring and practical. It's grounded in the latest evidence-based science—from mitochondrial health and telomere preservation to gut optimization, detoxification, sleep, movement, and more. You'll discover the top longevity foods, essential nutraceuticals, and cutting-edge biohacking tools. But beyond the protocols, what you'll find in these pages is *hope*—a clear and compelling vision that your best years can still be ahead of you.

This book also speaks to the soul. The Osenis understand that longevity is not merely a biological process—it is a sacred promise. As Scripture reminds us, "With long life I will satisfy him and show him My salvation" (Psalm 91:16). Yes, the path to a vibrant life is paved with intention, education, and action—but it is also a spiritual calling. This book bridges that gap beautifully.

As someone who has walked this journey with thousands of patients—watching some fall to illness and others rise into radiant health, I know the power of choice. And if you're holding this book, you're ready to make that choice. To turn knowledge into practice. To transform your health, your energy, and your future.

Dr. Olusegun and Catherine Oseni have poured their hearts, their brilliance, and their mission into these pages. So read it. Digest it. Share it. And above all—*live it.*

To your health, your vitality, and your legacy,

Jack Wolfson, DO

Cardiologist & Founder, Natural Heart Doctor

Author of *The Paleo Cardiologist: The Natural Way to Heart Health*

ENDORSEMENTS

"Aging is inevitable—but decline doesn't have to be. *HealthSpangevity*™ is a bold, science-rooted guide that redefines what it means to grow older. With actionable strategies, breakthrough insights, and a fresh perspective on vitality, this book flips the script on aging and empowers you to thrive at every stage of life. If you're ready to reclaim your energy, resilience, and purpose—and challenge the outdated narrative of inevitable decline—this is your blueprint. Inspiring, practical, and profoundly empowering, it's a must-read for anyone who wants to add not just years to their life, but life to their years."

Andie Crosby
President, Calroy Health Sciences

"As someone deeply immersed in the science of longevity, I've read countless books that overpromise and underdeliver. This isn't one of them. Drs. Oseni bring something rare and refreshing: depth without dogma, clarity without oversimplification. Their work is thoroughly researched, highly accessible, and refreshingly practical. They masterfully bridge the gap between cutting-edge science and real-life application, making this book not just informative, but truly transformative. If you're serious about living longer, healthier, and with greater purpose, this is the guide you'll want close at hand."

Suzanne Jeannette Ferree, MD, FAARM
Physician, Educator, Speaker, Author
Senior Physician at Vine Medical Associates

"As a longevity specialist and mentor committed to helping others extend both lifespan and healthspan, I find this book 'Healthspangevity™ to be a tour de force in personalized, science-backed wellness. Drs. Catherine and Olusegun Oseni have masterfully synthesized decades of clinical insight with the latest in functional and integrative medicine. This isn't just another health book, it's a comprehensive blueprint for reversing biological age, revitalizing cellular health, and reclaiming energy, purpose, and vitality at every stage of life. The concept of Healthspangevity™ is visionary, reminding us that growing older doesn't mean growing weaker—it means getting smarter, stronger, and more intentional about how we live.

What sets this work apart is its fusion of cutting-edge research with deeply humanistic care. From mitochondrial health to gut-brain optimization, from the power of hormesis to the art of biohacking, the Oseni team doesn't just inform—they empower. This book will inspire health professionals, biohackers, and everyday wellness seekers alike. If you're ready to age on your own terms—with energy, clarity, and joy—this book is your indispensable guide. I wholeheartedly recommend it to anyone seeking to live not only a long life but a meaningful one."

Dr. Mike Van Thielen, PhD.
PhD. Holistic Nutrition, Biohacking, and Longevity Expert
Founder of the Limitless Lab

"As the Director of the Centre for Heart & Vascular Health at the Heart Center of North Texas, I am constantly seeking comprehensive resources that can guide both patients and healthcare professionals toward optimal health and longevity.

"Healthspangevity™: Unlocking Longevity and Vitality" by Dr. Catherine Oseni and Dr. Olusegun Oseni is an exceptional addition to the field of integrative and functional medicine. This book is a meticulously crafted guide that delves into the science of aging, offering practical strategies to enhance healthspan and lifespan. The authors expertly blend cutting-edge research with actionable insights, making complex concepts accessible to a broad audience. From the importance of telomere preservation and mitochondrial function to the role of nutrition, exercise, and stress management, each chapter is a treasure trove of valuable information. Drs. Oseni's dedication to personalized medicine is evident throughout the book. Their emphasis on functional medicine testing and tailored interventions provides a roadmap for individuals to proactively manage their health. The inclusion of emerging therapies and innovative practices further underscores the book's relevance in today's rapidly evolving healthcare landscape. This book is a comprehensive wellness manual that empowers readers to take control of their health journey. It is an indispensable resource for anyone committed to living a longer, healthier, and more vibrant life. I highly recommend it to both patients and healthcare professionals seeking to enhance their understanding of longevity and vitality.

Stephen D. Newman, M.D., FACC, FAHA, FAS

“From the very first page, "Unlocking Longevity, Healthspan, and Vitality" stands out as a truly exceptional guide to living not just longer, but better. This book is a masterful blend of cutting-edge science, practical wisdom, and compassionate coaching-a rare combination that makes it both deeply informative and genuinely inspiring.

What I love most about this book is how it demystifies the science of aging, taking readers on a journey from the cellular level (like telomere preservation and mitochondrial health) all the way to the big-picture strategies for crafting a vibrant, resilient life. The chapters are thoughtfully organized, covering everything from nutrition, movement, and sleep, to the emerging frontiers of epigenetics, biohacking, and functional medicine testing. Each section is packed with actionable steps, clear explanations, and real-world examples that make even the most complex topics accessible.

The authors' passion for holistic health shines through every page. Their approach isn't about quick fixes or fads-it's about empowering readers to understand their own bodies, make informed choices, and build a personalized plan for lifelong vitality. I especially appreciate the focus on healthspan (not just lifespan), the integration of mental and emotional well-being, and the practical tools for tracking progress and adapting to life's changes.

Whether you're a health enthusiast, a practitioner, or simply someone who wants to take charge of your future, this book is must-read. It's the ultimate roadmap for anyone ready to unlock their potential and thrive at every age. I feel incredibly proud of my friends for creating such a comprehensive and empowering resource, and I can't recommend it highly enough!

To my brilliant friends: You've created a masterpiece that belongs on the shelves of every functional medicine clinic, biohacker's garage lab, and forward-thinking human's nightstand. This isn't a book-it's a legacy.

To everyone else: If you're ready to trade "aging gracefully" for dominating your biological destiny, grab this book immediately. Your 100-year-old self-will high-five you across time."

Sahar Swidan, Pharm.D., BCPS, ABAAHP, FAARFM, FACA
CEO, NeuroPharm
Adjunct Associate Professor, GWU School of Medicine
and Wayne State University

TABLE OF CONTENTS

ABOUT THE AUTHORS

Dr. Catherine Oseni, Pharm.D., FAAMFM, ABAAHP, FICT

Meet Dr. Catherine Oseni—a trailblazer in functional and integrative medicine, with nearly two decades of hands-on patient care. She is the Founder and CEO of Alpha Care Wellness Center, Director of Integrative Medicine at the Center for Cancer & Blood Disorders, and the creator of *Alphaceuticals by Dr. Catherine,* a nutraceutical line focused on vitality, hormone balance, and longevity.

Board-certified in Metabolic and Nutritional Medicine and a Fellow of the American Academy of Anti-Aging Medicine, Dr. Catherine specializes in hormone therapy, fertility support, integrative cancer care, and anti-aging protocols. She combines science-based therapies with holistic strategies to help patients thrive at every stage of life.

She co-leads The Oseni Institute alongside her husband, Dr. Olusegun Oseni. Together, they bring over 50 years of combined expertise to the forefront of functional and longevity medicine. Named one of Parker County's Most Extraordinary Women of 2023, Dr. Catherine's work continues to redefine health with purpose, compassion, and innovation.

Dr. Olusegun Oseni, M.D., FCCP, DABSM
CEO and Medical Director of Lung and Sleep Specialists of North Texas.

Dr. Olusegun Oseni isn't just a doctor; he's a wellness architect designing blueprints for longer, stronger, and more vibrant lives. As Medical Director of Alpha Care Wellness Center, Dr. Oseni brings a powerhouse combination of expertise in internal medicine, pulmonary care, critical care, and sleep medicine. His approach? Blend the best of modern medicine with integrative health strategies to help people feel unstoppable.

Dr. Oseni believes that true health goes beyond the absence of disease—it's about building a life filled with energy, resilience, and purpose. From tackling complex conditions like mold toxicity and Chronic Inflammatory Response Syndrome (CIRS) to optimizing sleep and metabolic health, he's dedicated to helping patients unlock their body's full potential. His vision is simple yet profound: empowering people to live long, vibrant lives with clarity, strength, and fulfillment.

Their Shared Mission:

Together, Dr. Catherine and Dr. Olusegun Oseni are revolutionizing the way we think about health and aging. Their mission is to empower individuals to break free from the cycle of symptom management and embrace a proactive, holistic approach to longevity and vitality. At Alpha Care Wellness Center, they combine cutting-edge science with personalized care to help people not just survive—but truly thrive.

Their vision is to create a world where health is more than a checklist; it's a dynamic, lifelong journey toward energy, resilience, and joy. Because living longer is good—but living longer and loving every moment? That's the ultimate goal.

INTRODUCTION

What is Healthspangevity™?

Healthspangevity™ (noun): The dynamic synergy between sustained peak performance and longevity, ensuring optimal vitality, resilience, and function throughout the aging process. It represents the intersection of healthspan (quality of life) and longevity (lifespan), emphasizing the ability to maintain strength, cognition, and overall well-being as we age.

Why Healthspangevity™?

Let's face it: we all want to live long—but what's the point of adding years to your life if those years aren't filled with vitality, purpose, and joy? Enter Healthspangevity™: the fusion of *healthspan* and *longevity*, a concept that's all about living longer and better. It's not just about stacking birthdays on your calendar; it's about celebrating each year with energy, clarity, and the ability to do what you love—without being weighed down by age-related decline.

Science has given us the means to extend our lifespan, but what about the quality of those extra years? While longevity measures the length of your life, healthspan focuses on how many of those years are spent in *good health—free from chronic disease, full of vitality, and thriving both physically and mentally*. Healthspangevity™ is the goal: optimizing both.

The Divine Blueprint for Longevity

"With long life I will satisfy him and show him my salvation." *(Psalms 91:16)*

Longevity is not just a modern aspiration—it's a divine promise. Throughout history, God has provided us with the knowledge and tools to live a long and vibrant life. Prayer, fasting, meditation, avoiding known dangers, and cultivating wisdom about the body's needs—these are all gifts designed to support optimal health and extended vitality. Yet, while these tools are available, every individual has a crucial role to play in their own health journey.

We've seen firsthand what happens when this responsibility is ignored. As intensivists working in the ICU, and as functional medicine doctors, we have treated countless elderly patients struggling with multiple organ failures—lives prolonged by modern medicine but diminished by preventable, age-related diseases. It doesn't have to be this way.

Imagine a world where your later years aren't spent managing disease but thriving with purpose. Picture celebrating your 100th birthday while still hiking, dancing, and mentoring the next generation. That's the promise of Healthspangevity™—and it's within your reach.

The Secret to Aging Well

Here's the truth: aging is inevitable, but how you age is your choice. Most of what we associate with aging—wrinkles, sluggishness, chronic disease—isn't dictated solely by genetics. It's driven by lifestyle. Your diet, movement, stress levels, sleep, and exposure to environmental toxins all influence your body's ability to stay strong and resilient.

This is where epigenetics comes in, proving that your genes are not your destiny. Your choices can flip genetic "switches" on or off, determining whether you thrive or succumb to disease. At the Oseni Institute, we've spent decades helping people rewrite their aging story—using functional medicine, integrative therapies, and cutting-edge longevity science.

Traditional medicine often waits until disease takes root before intervening. Our approach? Prevent it from taking root in the first place.

The Path to Healthspangevity™

Our mission is simple: to make Healthspangevity™ accessible to everyone. Whether it's optimizing your nutrition, upgrading your lifestyle, or embracing the latest breakthroughs in biohacking, this isn't just a theory—it's a way of life.

So, ask yourself:

- How can you reverse the clock on biological aging?
- How can you stay vibrant, fulfilled, and energized as you age?
- How can you ensure your golden years are truly golden?

The answers lie in Healthspangevity™.

Aging gracefully isn't a myth, it's a choice. Let's make it yours. The journey starts now.

"Don't just extend life—enrich it, enjoy it, and expand its possibilities."

Drs. Oseni

CHAPTER 1
AGING ACCELERATORS
How to slow cellular aging?

Aging. It's the one journey we're all on, whether we like it or not. From the moment we take our first breath, the biological clock starts ticking. At first, it's all about growth, energy, and boundless curiosity. But as the years roll by, things start to slow down. Joints creak, memory play hide-and-seek, and suddenly, your favorite jeans from a decade ago seem to have mysteriously shrunk.

So, what exactly is going on? Why does our once-springy, resilient body begin to lose its edge? The answer lies in a complex symphony of molecular, cellular, and systemic changes. Let's break it down in a way that won't put you to sleep (because, let's be honest, sleep is already one of those things we're struggling to get enough of as we age!).

The Science of Aging: A Slow but Steady Decline.

Aging is essentially a gradual, natural process where our physiological functions start to decline over time. This makes us more susceptible to diseases, weakens our physical and mental abilities, and ultimately, well... leads to the endgame. But before we get too grim, let's explore what's happening on different levels inside the body.

Cellular Aging: Where It All Begins

Cells are the tiny engines that keep our bodies running, but like any machine, they wear out. Here's how:

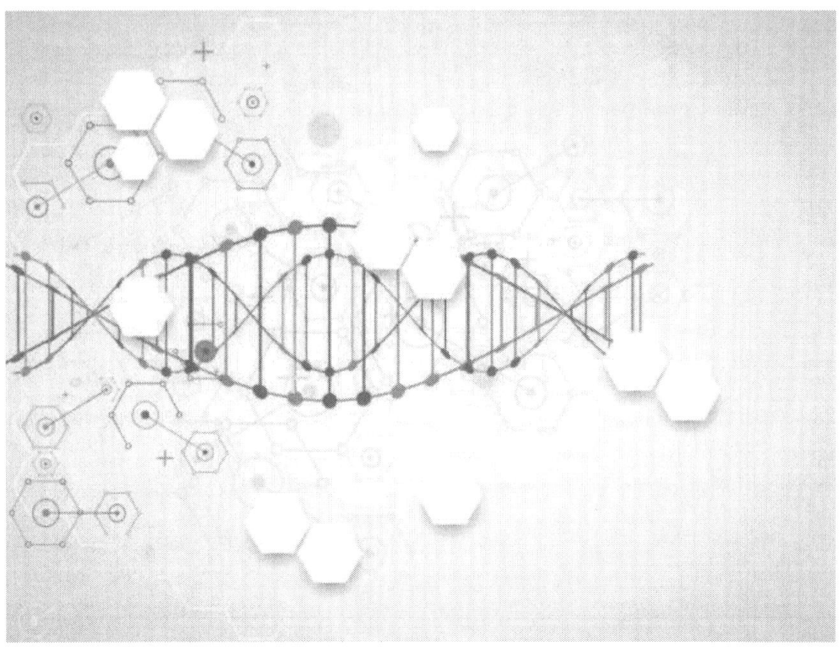

DNA Damage: Every day, our cells take a beating from environmental factors like UV rays, pollution, and even stress. This leads to DNA mutations and errors, which accumulate over time and contribute to aging.

Telomere Shortening: Think of telomeres as the little plastic caps on the ends of shoelaces. They protect our DNA, but every time a cell divides, these caps get a little shorter. When they wear down too much, cells lose their ability to function properly.

Mitochondrial Dysfunction: The mitochondria, aka the powerhouses of the cell, produces the energy we need to survive. But as we age, they become less efficient, leading to fatigue, muscle weakness, and even cognitive decline.

Systemic Aging: The Bigger Picture

While cells battle their microscopic struggles, the effects of aging become glaringly obvious at the whole-body level. Here are some telltale signs:

Muscle Loss (Sarcopenia): The days of effortlessly jumping out of bed? Gone. Muscle mass naturally declines, making us weaker and more prone to falls.

Metabolism Slows Down: That ice cream sundae you once burned off in an hour? Now it's setting up permanent residence on your waistline.

Cognitive Decline: Ever walked into a room and completely forgotten why? That's your brain playing tricks on you. Aging slows down neural communication, making memory and learning a bit trickier.

Weakened Immune System: The body's defense squad isn't as sharp as it used to be, which is why infections and diseases become more of a threat as we age.

The Aging Paradox: It's Not All Bad!

Before you resign yourself to a future of rocking chairs and early bedtimes, here's some good news: Aging isn't just about decline. There's wisdom, experience, and—if you play your cards right—plenty of ways to slow down the not-so-fun aspects of getting older.

Lifestyle choices like a nutrient-rich diet, regular movement (yes, even when the couch is calling), proper sleep, stress management, and cutting-edge wellness strategies (hello, molecular hydrogen!) can keep you feeling vibrant for years to come.

So, while aging may be inevitable, how you age is, to a large extent, up to you. Embrace the journey, fuel your body wisely, and remember—age is just a number, but energy and vitality? Those are things you can actively control.

Aging Accelerators and Biological Stressors

Certain factors accelerate the aging process and contribute to premature aging and age-related diseases. These are broadly categorized into biological stressors and lifestyle-related accelerators.

1. Oxidative Stress

Cause:

An imbalance between the production of reactive oxygen species (ROS) and the body's ability to neutralize them with antioxidants.

Impact:

ROS damage DNA, proteins, and lipids, contributing to cellular aging, inflammation, and chronic diseases like cancer and cardiovascular disease.

Prevention:

- Antioxidant-rich diets (berries, green tea, dark leafy greens)
- Regular physical activity in moderation
- Avoiding excessive sun exposure and smoking

2. Chronic Inflammation (Inflammaging)

Cause:

Persistent, low-grade inflammation due to poor diet, sedentary lifestyle, infections, and stress.

Impact:

Accelerates tissue damage, contributes to chronic diseases (arthritis, Alzheimer's, diabetes), and impairs immune function.

Prevention:

- Anti-inflammatory diets (omega-3s, turmeric, ginger)
- Stress management practices (meditation, deep breathing)
- Regular, moderate exercise

3. Telomere Shortening

Cause:

Telomeres, the protective caps on chromosomes, naturally shorten with each cell division. Accelerated by stress, poor diet, and smoking.

Impact:

Once telomeres become critically short, cells enter senescence or die, leading to tissue aging and disease susceptibility.

Prevention:

- Regular exercise (especially aerobics)
- Stress reduction techniques (yoga, mindfulness)
- Nutrient-rich diets high in antioxidants

Cause:

Telomeres, the protective caps on chromosomes, naturally shorten with each cell division. Accelerated by stress, poor diet, and smoking.

Impact:

Once telomeres become critically short, cells enter senescence or die, leading to tissue aging and disease susceptibility.

Prevention:

- Regular exercise (especially aerobics)
- Stress reduction techniques (yoga, mindfulness)
- Nutrient-rich diets high in antioxidants

4. Mitochondrial Dysfunction

Cause:

Mitochondria, the powerhouses of our cells, are responsible for generating ATP, the energy currency of life. However, several factors can impair their function:

Oxidative Stress: Excessive free radicals overwhelm the body's natural antioxidant defenses, leading to mitochondrial DNA (mtDNA) damage and impaired energy production.

Poor Diet: Processed foods, excessive sugar, and unhealthy fats promote inflammation, insulin resistance, and mitochondrial degradation.

Sedentary Lifestyle: A lack of physical activity leads to fewer and weaker mitochondria, reducing overall ATP output.

Environmental Toxins: Exposure to heavy metals, pesticides, and pollutants can damage mitochondrial membranes and impair function.

Aging: Natural mitochondrial decline occurs with age, but lifestyle choices can accelerate or slow this process.

Impact:

When mitochondria function poorly, energy production drops, and the entire body suffers. Common consequences include:

Chronic Fatigue: A hallmark symptom, as cells fail to generate sufficient ATP.

Neurodegeneration: Impaired mitochondria contribute to diseases like Alzheimer's, Parkinson's, and multiple sclerosis due to increased oxidative stress and cellular apoptosis.

Metabolic Disorders: Insulin resistance, obesity, and type 2 diabetes are linked to mitochondrial dysfunction.

Cardiovascular Disease: Poor mitochondrial efficiency affects heart cells, leading to increased risk of hypertension and heart failure.

Inflammation & Immune Dysfunction: A weakened immune system due to ATP shortages makes the body more vulnerable to infections and chronic diseases.

Prevention & Optimization:

The good news? Mitochondria are highly adaptable and can be rejuvenated with the right interventions.

Exercise for Mitochondrial Biogenesis:

- High-Intensity Interval Training (HIIT): Short bursts of intense exercise stimulate the production of new mitochondria and improve their efficiency.
- Endurance Training: Activities like running, cycling, and swimming enhance mitochondrial density and oxygen utilization.
- Resistance Training: Strength training promotes mitochondrial adaptations in muscle cells, boosting overall energy production.

Nutritional Support for Mitochondrial Health:

- Coenzyme Q10 (CoQ10): Essential for ATP production and acts as a powerful antioxidant protecting mitochondria.
- Magnesium: A critical cofactor in ATP production and energy metabolism.
- B Vitamins (B1, B2, B3, B6, B12): Play vital roles in the electron transport chain and mitochondrial energy production.
- Omega-3 Fatty Acids: Found in fish oil, they support mitochondrial membrane integrity and reduce inflammation.

- Polyphenols (Resveratrol, Quercetin, Curcumin): Plant compounds that activate mitochondrial biogenesis and protect against oxidative stress.

Metabolic Strategies to Boost Mitochondria:

- Intermittent Fasting: Promotes autophagy, allowing the body to recycle damaged mitochondria and stimulate the growth of new ones.
- Ketogenic Diet: Low-carb, high-fat diets encourage mitochondrial efficiency by shifting the body's primary energy source to ketones, which generate less oxidative stress.
- Cold Exposure & Heat Therapy: Ice baths, cryotherapy, and sauna sessions enhance mitochondrial function by inducing beneficial stress responses.

Lifestyle & Environmental Protection:

- Reduce Toxin Exposure: Minimize exposure to heavy metals (e.g., mercury, lead), air pollution, and pesticides that damage mitochondria.
- Optimize Sleep: Deep, restorative sleep is crucial for mitochondrial repair and detoxification.
- Stress Management: Chronic stress elevates cortisol, which impairs mitochondrial function—practices like meditation, breathwork, and nature exposure help maintain balance.

By optimizing mitochondrial function, we can significantly enhance energy levels, brain health, longevity, and overall vitality.

5. DNA Damage and Genomic Instability

Cause:

Environmental toxins (pollution, radiation), poor diet, and lifestyle factors cause DNA mutations and impair repair mechanisms.

Impact:

Increases the risk of cancer, accelerates tissue degeneration, and disrupts normal cell function.

Prevention:

- Avoid exposure to harmful chemicals and radiation
- Maintain a nutrient-dense diet (vitamins A, C, E, zinc)
- Adequate sleep for DNA repair

6. Cellular Senescence

Cause:

Cellular senescence occurs when cells become too damaged or stressed to function properly. Triggers include DNA damage, oxidative stress, telomere shortening, and chronic inflammation. Instead of dying off, these cells enter a state of permanent arrest where they stop dividing but refuse to leave.

Impact:

These "zombie cells" linger in tissues, releasing harmful pro-inflammatory chemicals known as the senescence-associated secretory phenotype (SASP). This toxic cocktail damages nearby healthy cells, promotes chronic inflammation, and accelerates aging. Over time, the accumulation of senescent cells contributes to age-related diseases like osteoarthritis, Alzheimer's, cardiovascular disease, and even cancer.

Prevention and Solutions:

- Natural senolytics: Certain natural compounds, like quercetin (found in apples, onions, and capers) and fisetin (found in strawberries and persimmons), have been shown to help clear out senescent cells.
- Regular Exercise: Moderate physical activity can reduce inflammation and slow the accumulation of senescent cells.
- Intermittent Fasting: Fasting activates autophagy, the body's natural cleanup process, which helps remove dysfunctional cells.
- Anti-Inflammatory Diet: Eating foods rich in antioxidants and healthy fats (like berries, leafy greens, and omega-3s) can lower chronic inflammation and limit senescent cell buildup.

Bottom Line: Clearing out these cellular freeloaders is crucial for maintaining healthy tissues and slowing down the aging process. Out with the old, in with the vibrant!

7. Glycation and Advanced Glycation End Products (AGEs)

Cause: Excessive sugar intake leads to glucose molecules binding to proteins and fats, forming AGEs.

Impact: AGEs stiffen tissues, damage collagen, and contribute to skin aging, diabetes, and cardiovascular disease.

Prevention:

- Limit intake of processed sugars and refined carbs
- Increase intake of antioxidants to neutralize AGEs
- Regular physical activity

8. Hormonal Imbalances

Cause:

Hormones are the body's biochemical messengers, regulating metabolism, mood, energy levels, muscle growth, immune function, and overall vitality. However, as we age, key hormones naturally decline, leading to widespread physiological changes. Factors contributing to hormonal imbalances include:

Aging: Declining levels of growth hormone, testosterone, estrogen, progesterone, and DHEA.

Chronic Stress: Elevated cortisol disrupts hormone production, suppressing beneficial hormones like testosterone and progesterone.

Nutrient Deficiencies: Poor diet lacking in essential fats, vitamins, and minerals impairs hormone synthesis.

Lack of Physical Activity: Sedentary lifestyles contribute to lower levels of growth hormone, testosterone, and insulin sensitivity.

Environmental Toxins & Endocrine Disruptors: Chemicals like BPA, Phthalates, and pesticides interfere with natural hormone production and balance.

Poor Sleep Patterns: Inadequate sleep disrupts circadian rhythms and impairs hormone regulation.

Key Hormones Affected & Their Role:

Testosterone (Men & Women): Essential for muscle mass, fat metabolism, energy, and libido. Declining levels lead to fatigue, weight gain, and reduced cognitive function.

Estrogen (Women): Supports bone density, brain function, and cardiovascular health. Low estrogen contributes to osteoporosis, cognitive decline, and mood disorders.

Progesterone (Women): Balances estrogen, supports sleep, mood, and immune regulation. Declining levels contribute to anxiety, insomnia, and auto-immune susceptibility.

Growth Hormone (GH): Crucial for cellular repair, fat metabolism, muscle growth, and energy production. Declines with age, leading to increased fat storage and reduced vitality.

DHEA (Dehydroepiandrosterone): Precursor to testosterone and estrogen, supports immune function, brain health, and resilience to stress.

Thyroid Hormones: Regulate metabolism, energy levels, and temperature control. Imbalances can lead to weight gain, fatigue, and depression.

Insulin: Controls blood sugar levels. Insulin resistance due to hormonal imbalance can lead to diabetes and metabolic disorders.

Cortisol: While necessary for stress response, chronic elevation disrupts other hormones, leading to fatigue, weight gain, and immune suppression.

Impact:

Hormonal imbalances disrupt nearly every system in the body, leading to a cascade of negative effects:

Metabolic Dysfunction:

- Increased fat storage, especially visceral fat
- Reduced ability to build and maintain lean muscle
- Increased risk of obesity and type 2 diabetes

Cognitive Decline & Mood Disorders:

- Brain fog, memory loss, and difficulty concentrating
- Increased risk of anxiety, depression, and mood swings
- Poor sleep quality due to progesterone and melatonin imbalances

Increased Risk of Autoimmune Diseases

- Hormones regulate immune function—imbalances can lead to excessive immune responses, increasing susceptibility to autoimmune diseases like rheumatoid arthritis, lupus, Hashimoto's thyroiditis, and multiple sclerosis.
- Low progesterone and estrogen fluctuations contribute to immune overactivity and chronic inflammation.
- Cortisol dysregulation weakens immune tolerance, leading to increased auto-antibody production.

Cardiovascular Risks:

- Low estrogen increases the risk of heart disease and arterial stiffness.
- Imbalanced cortisol and insulin levels contribute to hypertension and cholesterol imbalances.

Reproductive & Sexual Dysfunction:

- Decreased libido in both men and women
- Erectile dysfunction in men due to low testosterone
- Irregular menstrual cycles and menopause-related symptoms in women

Bone & Joint Health Decline:

- Estrogen and progesterone are crucial for bone density—declines leading to osteoporosis.
- Low testosterone contributes to joint pain and muscle weakness.

<u>Prevention & Hormonal Optimization:</u>

Hormone levels can be optimized naturally through targeted lifestyle interventions:

<u>Exercise for Hormonal Balance:</u>

- Strength Training & Resistance Workouts: Increases testosterone, growth hormone, and insulin sensitivity.
- High-Intensity Interval Training (HIIT): Boosts growth hormone and improves metabolic function.

- Yoga & Stress-Reduction Exercises: Helps balance cortisol and improves progesterone and estrogen regulation.

Nutritional Strategies for Hormone Production:

- Healthy Fats:
    - Cholesterol is the building block of hormones—consume avocados, olive oil, coconut oil, grass-fed butter, and fatty fish.
    - Omega-3 fatty acids reduce inflammation and support hormone synthesis.

- Protein Intake:
    - Essential amino acids support growth hormone and testosterone production.
    - Include sources like grass-fed meats, wild-caught fish, eggs, and plant-based proteins.
- Nutrient-Rich Foods:
    - Magnesium & Zinc: Support testosterone and progesterone production (found in nuts, seeds, dark chocolate, and leafy greens).
    - Vitamin D: Crucial for testosterone, estrogen, and immune function (sunlight exposure and foods like salmon and mushrooms).
    - B Vitamins: Important for energy metabolism and hormone synthesis (found in eggs, beef liver, and whole grains).

Lifestyle Strategies to Regulate Hormones:

- Prioritize Sleep:
    - Deep, restorative sleep (7-9 hours) regulates growth hormone, testosterone, and cortisol.

    - Avoid blue light before bedtime and maintain a consistent sleep schedule.
- Manage Stress & Cortisol Levels:
    - Meditation, breathwork, and nature exposure lower cortisol and improve hormonal resilience.
    - Adaptogenic herbs like ashwagandha and rhodiola help balance stress responses.
- Optimize Gut Health:
    - The gut microbiome influences hormone metabolism—consume probiotic-rich foods (fermented vegetables, kefir, yogurt) to support hormonal regulation.

Intermittent Fasting & Metabolic Health:

- Short fasting windows (12-16 hours) can improve insulin sensitivity, boost growth hormone, and support cellular repair.
- Help balance estrogen and testosterone levels while reducing inflammation.

Minimize Endocrine Disruptors:

- Avoid plastics, BPA, and synthetic chemicals in food containers and personal care products.
- Choose organic produce and hormone-free animal products to reduce exposure to xenoestrogens.

Consider Hormone Replacement Therapy (HRT) if Necessary:

- Bioidentical Hormone Therapy (BHRT): A natural approach to replacing declining hormones in a balanced manner.

- DHEA & Progesterone Supplementation: Can support immune health, reduce inflammation, and enhance sleep quality.
- Always consult with a qualified healthcare professional for personalized hormone optimization.

Conclusion:

Hormonal balance is the foundation of health, energy, and longevity. By proactively supporting hormone production through strength training, proper nutrition, quality sleep, and stress management, we can mitigate age-related hormonal decline and maintain peak physical and cognitive function.

9. Environmental and Lifestyle Stressors

Key Contributors:

Chronic Psychological Stress: Persistent mental and emotional strain elevates cortisol levels.

Poor Sleep Habits: Inconsistent or inadequate sleep disrupts the body's repair and recovery processes.

Sedentary Behavior: Prolonged inactivity weakens muscles, slows metabolism, and accelerates aging.

Exposure to Environmental Toxins: Pollutants, heavy metals, and chemicals can damage cells and organs, increasing oxidative stress.

Impact:

Continuous exposure to environmental and lifestyle stressors leads to elevated cortisol levels, fueling chronic inflammation and weakening the immune system. Over time, this accelerates the aging process, increasing the risk of diseases like diabetes, heart disease, and cognitive decline.

Prevention Strategies:

Adopt Mind-Body Practices: Engage in stress-reducing activities like meditation, deep breathing exercises, yoga, or Tai Chi to lower cortisol levels and enhance mental resilience.

Prioritize Quality Sleep: Aim for 7-9 hours of consistent, restorative sleep each night to allow the body to repair and regenerate.

Minimize Toxin Exposure: Improve indoor air quality with air purifiers, choose organic or whole foods to reduce chemical intake, and use natural household products.

Stay Physically Active: Incorporate daily movement, even in small amounts, take walking breaks, stretch regularly, and avoid prolonged sitting.

1.1. Slowing Cellular Ageing

Cellular aging is the ultimate game of wear and tear, but on a microscopic level. Imagine each of your cells as a bustling factory working 24/7 to keep you alive and thriving. Over time, these factories slow down, parts start breaking, and efficiency plummets. This gradual decline in cell function is driven by accumulated damage from oxidative stress, DNA mutations, and faltering repair mechanisms.

Eventually, some cells wave the white flag, entering a state called senescence—where they stop dividing, become dysfunctional, and wreak havoc by releasing inflammatory signals. This cellular chaos contributes to tissue degeneration, wrinkles, and age-related diseases. Fun, right?

Strategies for Slowing Cellular Aging:

1.1.1. Telomere Preservation: Keep Your Shoelaces Intact

Activate Telomerase: While telomerase activation in humans is still under study, lifestyle habits like regular exercise and a Mediterranean diet have been shown to support telomere health.

Nutritional Support: Vitamins C and E, polyphenols, and omega-3 fatty acids protect telomeres. Think berries, green tea, and walnuts!

Stress Reduction: Chronic stress accelerates telomere shortening. Yoga, meditation, and deep breathing are your allies.

1.3.2. Enhancing Antioxidant Defenses: Armor Up!

Antioxidant-Rich Diet: Fill your plate with colorful fruits and veggies. Blueberries, spinach, and nuts are your best friends.

Supplement Wisely: Boost your defenses with CoQ10, alpha-lipoic acid, and glutathione.

Exercise Regularly: Physical activity enhances natural antioxidant production. Just avoid overtraining!

1.3.3. Supporting Mitochondrial Function: Power Up

Mitochondrial Biogenesis: Practices like moderate intensity training, HIIT (high intensity interval training), fasting, and cold exposure trigger the creation of new, healthy mitochondria.

Targeted Nutrients: pyrroloquinoline quinone (PQQ), acetyl-L-carnitine, and omega-3s can revitalize mitochondria.

Reduce Toxins: Cut back on processed foods and environmental toxins to lighten the load on your mitochondria.

1.3.4. Clearing Senescent Cells: Out with the Old

Senolytics: Compounds like quercetin and fisetin target and clear senescent cells.

Autophagy Activation: Fasting and regular exercise stimulates autophagy, your body's natural cleaning system.

Anti-Inflammatory Diet: Omega-3s, turmeric, and leafy greens can curb inflammation.

1.3.5. DNA Repair and Epigenetic Support: Guard Your Blueprint

DNA Repair Nutrients: Folate, B vitamins, NAD+ and zinc support DNA repair.

Epigenetic Modulation: Diet, exercise, and stress management influence gene expression in your favor.

1.4. The Impact of Slowing Cellular Aging on Healthspangevity™

1. Extended Healthspan and Lifespan:

Slow aging means more years of vibrant health, not just living longer but living better.

2. Improved Physical and Cognitive Function:

Healthier cells mean sharper minds, stronger bodies, and better mobility.

3. Lower Risk of Chronic Diseases:

Reducing cellular damage decreases the risk of heart disease, diabetes, and dementia.

4. Enhanced Resilience and Recovery:

Your body bounces back faster from stress, illness, and injury.

5. Better Mood and Emotional Well-being:

More energy and less pain led to a brighter, more positive outlook on life.

Aging is inevitable, but how your age is up to you. By protecting your cells, nurturing your mitochondria, and clearing out the cellular clutter, you can defy the usual script of aging. Imagine decades of energy, strength, and mental clarity, now that's a future worth investing in!

CHAPTER 2
THE FOUNDATIONS OF HEALTHSPANGEVITY

Welcome to the World of Healthspangevity™: Where Everything Is Connected!

Let's be honest—our bodies are like a high-tech, all-inclusive resort where every department needs to work in perfect harmony for the whole operation to thrive. Your digestive system? Oh, it's not just some food processor churning out energy; it's the control center influencing your immune defense, brainpower, and even your mood swings (yes, that hangry feeling is real!). And your heart? It's more than just a mechanical pump—it's a drama queen that reacts to stress, diet, and even the rollercoaster of your relationships. Break its rhythm, and it's sure to let you know!

In this chapter, we're diving deep into how these intricate systems are all tangled together in one big, beautiful web of health. Functional medicine isn't about slapping a Band-Aid on symptoms—it's about looking at the full picture. We'll explore how small shifts in one area—like ditching processed snacks for real food or finally tackling that stress monster—can create powerful ripple effects across your entire body. It's time to unlock the secrets of how your body really works and discover how these connections hold the key to not just living longer but living stronger. Buckle up, because your journey to mastering Healthspangevity™ starts now!

2 .1. Pillars of Longevity

The foundation of *Healthspangevity™* rests firmly on four essential pillars: Nutrition, Movement, Sleep, and Stress Management. These pillars are not merely components of a healthy lifestyle, they are the core drivers of long-term vitality, resilience, and disease prevention. Each one works synergistically to support the body's natural ability to heal, adapt, and thrive as we age. In this chapter, we'll explore how optimizing these pillars can unlock the key to living not only a longer life but a richer, more vibrant one.

Nutrition is far more than calories counting or following fleeting diet trends. It's about fueling your body with the right balance of macronutrients and micronutrients to nourish your cells, support metabolic processes, and combat inflammation. Food is both information and medicine—what you eat has the power to either protect you from chronic diseases or accelerate their onset. Understanding the relationship between nutrition and longevity allows you to make intentional choices that sustain your energy, mental clarity, and overall vitality.

Movement is the engine of longevity. Our bodies are designed for motion, and physical activity is essential for preserving muscle mass, protecting cardiovascular health, and supporting cognitive function. From strength training and aerobic conditioning to flexibility and mobility work, a balanced approach to movement ensures that your body remains strong, agile, and resilient against the physical challenges of aging. Movement isn't just about fitness, it's about maintaining independence, preventing injury, and enhancing your quality of life.

Sleep is the often-overlooked pillar that quietly governs nearly every aspect of health. It is during sleep that the body repairs tissues, consolidates memories, balances hormones, and strengthens the immune system. Poor sleep doesn't just lead to fatigue—it disrupts metabolic health, accelerates aging, and weakens mental resilience. Understanding the science of sleep and aligning your habits with your body's natural circadian rhythms is critical for long-term health and cognitive performance.

Stress Management is the linchpin that holds the other pillars together. Chronic stress silently undermines health by increasing inflammation, disrupting hormone balance, and accelerating aging. Left unchecked, it can unravel even the most disciplined health routines. Managing stress effectively means more than simply relaxing—it involves building mental resilience, regulating emotional responses, and creating sustainable habits that support a calm, balanced mind. Recognizing the profound connection between emotional well-being and physical health is essential for achieving longevity.

Together, these four pillars form a powerful framework for lifelong health. By understanding and strengthening each of them, you can create a resilient foundation that supports not only a longer lifespan but a more fulfilling and vibrant healthspan.

2.2. Epigenetics: Rewriting the Story of Aging and Longevity

What if I told you that your genes aren't the strict, unchangeable blueprint you were handed at birth, but more like a flexible script—complete with footnotes, edits, and even plot twists? Welcome to the world of *epigenetics*, where your daily choices, environment, and even your mindset play the role of editor-in-chief, deciding which parts of your genetic story get published and which stay in the drafts folder.

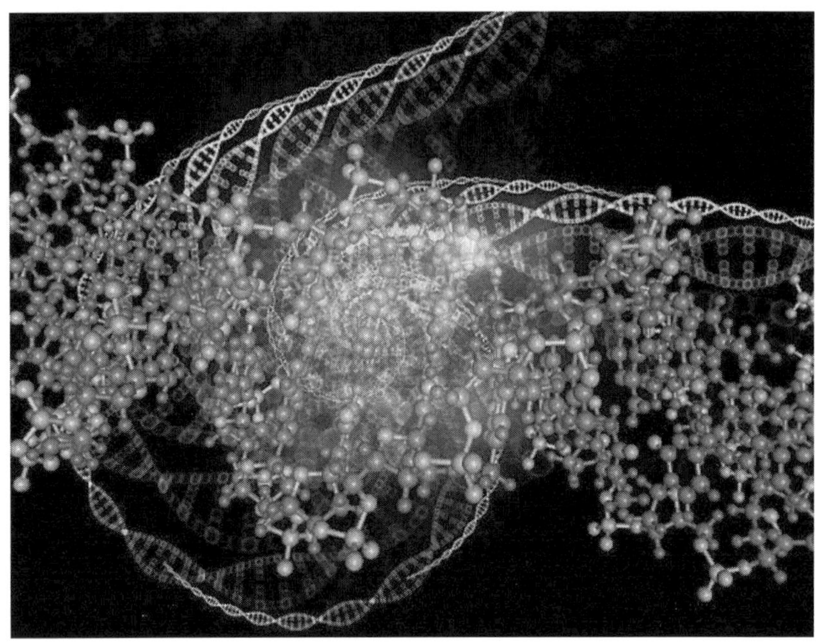

2.2.1. Genes vs. Epigenetics: Who's Really in Charge?

Let's clear something up: your DNA isn't your destiny. Yes, your genes provide the instruction manual for how your body operates, but epigenetics decides which instructions get followed. Imagine your DNA as a massive cookbook. Epigenetics is the head chef, choosing which recipes to whip up and which ones to ignore. Just because your family history includes heart disease or diabetes doesn't mean you're doomed to follow the same path. The chef can choose healthier recipes—and that chef is YOU.

2.2.1. The Epigenetic Switchboard

At the core of epigenetics are chemical tags—think of them as sticky notes on your DNA—that signal which genes should be turned on or off. These molecular switches are influenced by everything from your diet and exercise to stress and sleep. Smoking, poor diet, chronic stress? They slap on sticky notes that say, "Activate disease mode."

Meanwhile, a balanced diet, regular exercise, and meditation? Those add notes like, "Activate repair and longevity mode."

One of the main mechanisms behind this genetic editing is DNA methylation, where tiny methyl groups attach to your DNA, turning genes on or off.

Then there are histone modifications, which control how tight DNA is wound. Tightly wound DNA can hide genes, while loosely wound DNA makes them easily accessible. It's like managing a library where certain books (genes) are put on display, while others are locked away in storage.

2.2.2. Epigenetics and Aging: The Clock You Can Reset

Here's where things get interesting: aging isn't just about the years passing by, it's about how your genes are expressed over time. Enter the concept of the epigenetic clock, a tool scientists use to measure biological age based on DNA methylation patterns. Spoiler alert: your biological age doesn't always match your calendar age. You could be 50 but have the biological age of 35—or vice versa.

So, can you turn back the hands of this clock? Absolutely! Studies show that lifestyle changes can reverse biological aging. A groundbreaking study found that a plant-rich diet, regular exercise, stress reduction, and proper sleep *reversed* participants' biological age by up to three years—in just eight weeks! Imagine that: eight weeks to start rewriting your aging story.

2.2.3. Lifestyle as Gene Therapy (No Lab Required)

Let's talk about how you can biohack your genes for a longer, healthier life without needing a PhD in molecular biology. We simply implement the pillars we discussed earlier in this chapter:

1. Nutrition: Your fork is mightier than your DNA. Foods rich in polyphenols (like blueberries, green tea, and turmeric) can positively influence gene expression. Leafy greens and cruciferous veggies support methylation—a fancy way of saying they help turn on the good genes.

2. Exercise: Moving your body doesn't just make you fit your genes. Exercise activates genes that improve metabolism, repair cells, and even grow new brain cells. Sitting, on the other hand, tells your genes, "We're going downhill."

3. Stress Management: Chronic stress isn't just a mental drain—it changes your gene expression. Practices like meditation and deep breathing turn off genes linked to inflammation and disease. It's like flipping your internal switch from "panic" to "peace."

4. Sleep: Sleep is when your body does its best editing. Poor sleep disrupts DNA repair, while quality sleep supports gene activity that slows aging. In short, sleep like your life depends on it—because it does.

2.2.4. Can You Inherit Epigenetic Changes? (Thanks, Grandma)

Here's a plot twist: some epigenetic changes can be passed down to future generations. Studies on famine survivors showed that their grandchildren had altered gene expression related to metabolism and disease risk. So, your lifestyle choices today don't just impact you, they can echo through generations. Talk about family legacy!

But the reverse is also true. By making positive changes now, you can potentially break harmful cycles and pass on a genetic advantage. You're not just rewriting your story—you're editing the entire family saga.

2.2.5. The Future of Epigenetics: Aging on Your Own Terms

The future of aging may not lie in miracle pills but in understanding and optimizing our gene expression. Scientists are exploring epigenetic therapies that could one day prevent or even reverse age-related diseases. But until then, the most powerful tool is in your hands.

Your genes might load the gun, but your lifestyle pulls the trigger—or better yet, puts the safety on. So, why not start flipping those genetic switches in your favor?

In the grand story of your life, epigenetics hand you the pen. What kind of ending do you want to write?

2.3. Biohacking: Redefining the Path to Longevity

Imagine having the ability to upgrade your body and mind the way you update your smartphone. That's the essence of *biohacking*—the art and science of optimizing your biology to improve health, performance, and longevity. It's about taking control of your body's systems through strategic interventions, ranging from cutting-edge technology to simple lifestyle tweaks. In other words, biohacking is self-improvement on a cellular level.

2.3.1. What is Biohacking?

Biohacking is the practice of making small, incremental changes to your diet, lifestyle, and environment to improve your overall well-being. It's a personalized, data-driven approach to health that empowers individuals to enhance their physical and mental performance. Biohackers use science-backed strategies to "hack" biological processes and push the limits of human potential.

Biohacking methods range from simple practices—like adjusting sleep habits and nutrition—to more advanced techniques involving wearable technology, nootropics, genetic testing, and even stem cell therapy. Whether it's intermittent fasting, cold exposure, or using blue light blockers, every action aims to fine-tune the body's systems for peak performance and longevity.

2.3.2. Biohacking's Role in Longevity

So, how does biohacking extend your lifespan and, more importantly, your *healthspan*? By targeting the root causes of aging and chronic diseases, biohacking helps slow down biological aging and enhances the body's natural repair mechanisms.

1. Cellular Optimization: Techniques like intermittent fasting and autophagy-activating diets encourage the body to repair and recycle damaged cells, reducing inflammation and oxidative stress, two major drivers of aging.

2. Hormonal Balance: Biohacking strategies, such as sleep optimization and stress management, help regulate hormone levels. Balanced hormones support everything from metabolism to cognitive function, keeping the body resilient and youthful.

3. Mitochondrial Health: Mitochondria are the powerhouse of cells. Biohacking practices like molecular hydrogen, red light therapy, and targeted supplementation enhance mitochondrial function, boosting energy production and slowing cellular aging.

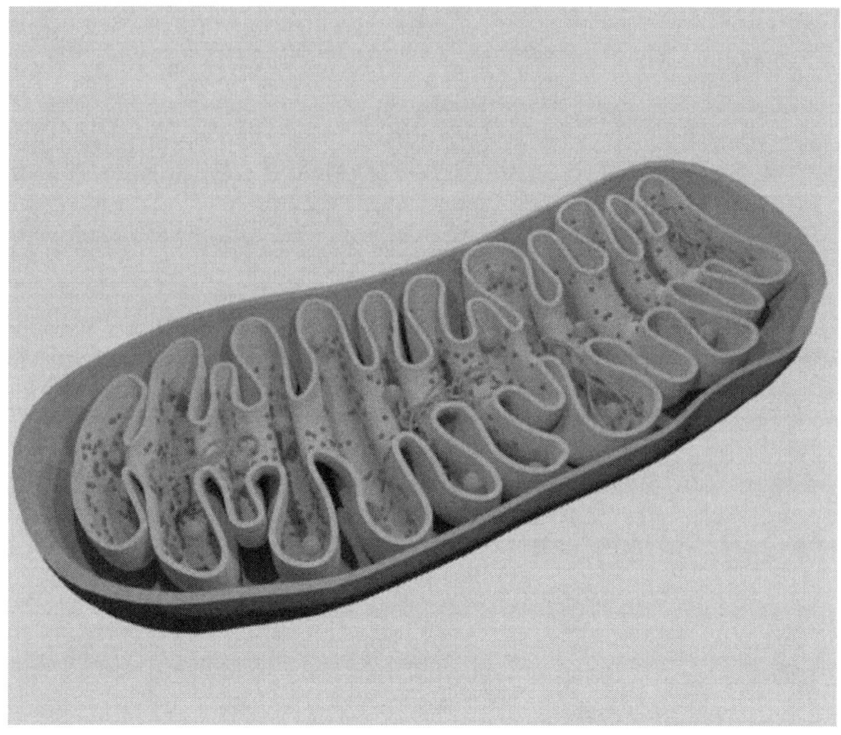

4. Genetic Expression: Biohackers use epigenetic insights to influence gene expression. Lifestyle changes, such as nutrient-rich diets and mindfulness practices, can activate genes that promote longevity and suppress those linked to disease.

5. Stress Adaptation: Chronic stress accelerates aging, but biohacking tools like meditation apps, heart rate variability (HRV) monitors, and adaptogenic herbs help build resilience and reduce the harmful effects of stress.

2.3.3. The Future of Biohacking and Longevity

As science advances, so does biohacking. Emerging technologies like CRISPR gene editing, stem cell regeneration, and personalized medicine are pushing the boundaries of human longevity. However, the foundation of biohacking remains rooted in understanding and working with your body's natural systems.

Biohacking empowers you to become the CEO of your own health. By combining ancient wisdom with modern science, you can make informed decisions that enhance your lifespan and, more importantly, the quality of your years. After all, what's the point of living longer if you're not living better?

In the journey toward longevity, biohacking isn't just a trend, it's a revolution. And the best part? You're in control

2.4. Setting the Stage - Initial Assessments and Health Baselines

Welcome to the starting line of your *Healthspangevity*™ journey! You wouldn't set off on a road trip without checking your gas tank, tires, and maybe Googling how far your destination is, right? The same goes for optimizing your health. Before you can supercharge your longevity and unlock your inner superhero, you need to know exactly where you stand. And no, "feeling fine" doesn't cut it—we're talking data, science, and some hardcore truth bombs about your body's current state.

2.4.1 Why Health Baselines Matter (Spoiler: They're Your Roadmap to Success)

Imagine trying to improve your finances without knowing how much is in your bank account. It's a guessing game that rarely ends well. Your health works the same way. Establishing solid health baselines gives you a crystal-clear picture of what's working, what's lagging, and what needs a serious intervention. Without these insights, you're basically throwing spaghetti (or kale) at the wall and hoping something sticks.

2.4.2. Meet Your Body's Dashboard: Key Biomarkers of Aging

Here's where we get into the nitty-gritty. These are the vital signs of how gracefully—or not—you're aging. Think of these as the warning lights on your car's dashboard. Ignore them, and you could end up stranded on the side of the road.

- Inflammation Markers (High Sensitivity CRP, IL-6): Chronic inflammation is the sneaky villain behind most age-related diseases. High levels? Time to fight the fire.
- Hormone Levels (Testosterone, Estrogen, Cortisol, DHEA-S. Progesterone, SHBG, Thyroid): Hormones are your body's text messages. If they're out of whack, your body isn't getting the right messages.
- Metabolic Health Indicators (Glucose, Insulin, Cholesterol, Lipoprotein (a), APO A, APO B): These numbers reveal how efficiently your body turns food into fuel and how well it manages energy storage. Spoiler: insulin resistance is not your friend.
- Oxidative Stress (Glutathione, CoQ10): This measures how well your body fights off cellular damage. Higher stress = faster aging.

2.4.3. Functional Medicine Assessments: Your Personalized Health Detective Work

Forget one-size-fits-all checkups. Functional medicine digs deeper to uncover the *why* behind your health challenges. It's like hiring a detective to solve the case of why you're tired, foggy, or just not feeling your best.

- Comprehensive Blood Panels: Not your basic "looks fine" bloodwork. We're talking in-depth nutrient profiles, thyroid panels, inflammatory markers, and more.
- Genetic Testing: Your genes are not your destiny, but they do offer clues. Genetic testing can reveal predispositions to certain diseases, how you metabolize nutrients, and how your body responds to stress.
- Lifestyle Analysis: Sleep habits, stress levels, diet, exercise, and even how much sunlight you get—these lifestyle factors directly influence how you age.

Tracking Progress: The Power of Measurable Results

Let's be honest—seeing results is motivating. Establishing health baselines isn't just a one-and-done deal. It's a roadmap, a before-and-after snapshot that shows how far you've come. Regular check-ins with these biomarkers help you adjust your strategies and celebrate your wins.

- Quarterly or Biannual Testing: Health isn't static. Regular testing keeps you ahead of potential issues and ensures you're trending in the right direction.
- Wearable Tech and Apps: Track your sleep, heart rate variability (HRV), steps, and even stress levels. Yes, your smartwatch can help you live longer!
- Symptom Tracking: How you *feel* is important too. Logging your energy levels, digestion, mood, and sleep can reveal patterns data alone can't show.

Know Thyself: The Ultimate Longevity Hack

Here's the truth: you can't change what you don't measure. Knowing your health baselines empowers you to take targeted action. Instead of guessing which diet, workout, or supplement might work, you'll know exactly what your body needs.

So, let's ditch the guesswork and embrace the data. It's time to take a hard (but loving) look under the hood, fine-tune the engine, and get ready for the drive of your life. Your body will thank you—and so will future you.

Buckle up. The road to optimal health and longevity starts *now*.

CHAPTER 3 NUTRITIONAL STRATEGIES FOR LONGEVITY

When it comes to unlocking the secrets of longevity, nutrition is the foundation of vibrant health and graceful aging. The intricate relationship between what we eat and how we age influences every aspect of our well-being, from cellular health to mental clarity. By integrating ancient wisdom, functional medicine principles, and modern dietary science, we can create a comprehensive roadmap to extend both lifespan and healthspan.

The Foundation: Food as Medicine

Food is more than sustenance; it's a potent modulator of our biology. Every bite we take acts as a biochemical signal, influencing gene expression, inflammation levels, hormone balance, and even the gut microbiome. Whole, nutrient-dense foods fuel vital functions, support cellular repair, and bolster resilience against disease. Conversely, diets laden with refined sugars, artificial additives, and inflammatory fats disrupt our physiological equilibrium and accelerate aging. Functional medicine underscores the importance of food as a cornerstone for restoring balance, vitality, and optimal health.

3.1. Core Principles of Longevity Nutrition

3.1.1. Macronutrient Balancing: The Power Trio

To build a robust foundation for health, it's essential to balance macronutrients—carbohydrates, proteins, and fats:

Carbohydrates: Complex carbohydrates from sources like quinoa, legumes, sweet potatoes, and whole grains provide sustained energy and fiber to support gut health. Refined sugars and processed carbs, however, accelerate aging by fueling inflammation and oxidative stress.

Proteins: Proteins are indispensable for muscle maintenance, immune function, and cellular repair. Opting for lean, high-quality sources such as wild-caught fish, grass-fed meats, eggs, and plant-based options like lentils and quinoa. Older adults benefit from increased protein intake to prevent sarcopenia (age-related muscle loss).

Fats: Healthy fats are crucial for brain function, heart health, and reducing inflammation. Prioritize monounsaturated and polyunsaturated fats from avocados, olive oil, nuts, seeds, and fatty fishlike salmon. Avoid trans fats and processed oils, which exacerbate cellular damage.

A macronutrient ratio of 40% complex carbs, 30% healthy fats, and 30% lean proteins supports balanced energy levels, hormonal harmony, and cellular longevity.

3.1.2. Anti-Inflammatory Eating: Combatting the Silent Killer

Chronic inflammation is a driving force behind most age-related diseases, including heart disease, Alzheimer's, and cancer. An anti-inflammatory diet acts as your armor against this silent threat. Incorporate foods rich in antioxidants, omega-3 fatty acids, and anti-inflammatory compounds:

- Fatty Fish: Salmon, mackerel, and sardines are rich in EPA and DHA, powerful anti-inflammatory omega-3s.

- Leafy Greens: Spinach, kale, and Swiss chard provide a wealth of vitamins, minerals, and fiber.
- Berries: Blueberries, strawberries, and blackberries are antioxidant powerhouses.
- Nuts and Seeds: Almonds, walnuts, chia seeds, and flaxseeds deliver healthy fats and fiber.
- Herbs and Spices: Turmeric (enhanced with black pepper), ginger, cinnamon, and garlic reduce inflammation and add depth to your meals.

The more colorful your plate, the greater the variety of anti-aging nutrients you'll consume. Aim for a vibrant "rainbow diet" to maximize your intake of phytonutrients.

3.1.3. Phytochemicals and Antioxidants: Nature's Defense System

Plants are nature's pharmacy, offering a wide array of phytochemicals and antioxidants to combat oxidative stress primary driver of aging. Key nutrients include:

Vitamin C: Found in citrus fruits, bell peppers, and broccoli, this vitamin is essential for collagen synthesis and cellular repair.

Vitamin E: Abundant in nuts, seeds, and avocados, it protects cells from free radical damage.

Polyphenols: Present in green tea, dark chocolate, and red wine, these compounds reduce inflammation and support cardiovascular health.

Carotenoids: Beta-carotene (carrots), lutein (spinach), and lycopene (tomatoes) enhance skin health, vision, and cellular resilience.

Snack on berries and nuts, sip green tea, and drizzle olive oil over your vegetables to harness these protective compounds.

3.2. Advanced Longevity Practices

3.2.1. Caloric Restriction and Intermittent Fasting

Reducing caloric intake while maintaining nutrient density has been linked to extended lifespan and enhanced cellular health. Intermittent fasting (IF) is an approachable method to achieve these benefits. Popular IF strategies include:

Time-Restricted Eating (TRE): Consuming all meals within an 8–10-hour window and fasting for the remaining hours.

5:2 Diet: Eating normally for five days a week and restricting calorie intake (~500-600 calories) on two non-consecutive days.

Fasting-Mimicking Diet (FMD): he **Fasting-Mimicking Diet (FMD)** is a structured, low-calorie, plant-based nutritional protocol designed to simulate the physiological effects of fasting while still providing essential nutrients. Developed by Dr. Valter Longo, this five-day dietary approach allows individuals to experience the benefits of prolonged fasting—such as cellular repair, metabolic optimization, and longevity—without the extreme deprivation associated with water-only fasting.

<u>How FMD Works:</u>

FMD strategically reduces calorie intake while maintaining specific macronutrient ratios to prevent the body from detecting food abundance. This keeps the body in a fasting-like metabolic state while still supplying essential nutrients.

Duration: Typically followed for five consecutive days per cycle.

Caloric Intake: Around 800–1,100 calories per day, depending on the protocol.

Macronutrient Breakdown:

- Low protein (to suppress IGF-1 and mTOR, reducing aging-related pathways)
- Low carbohydrates (to maintain ketosis and stabilize blood sugar)
- High healthy fats (to provide sustained energy while keeping insulin levels low)

<u>Biological Mechanisms Activated by FMD:</u>

By mimicking a fasted state, FMD triggers key longevity pathways that enhance cellular resilience, repair, and overall health:

<u>Sirtuin Activation (SIRT1 & SIRT3):</u>

- Sirtuins are longevity-promoting enzymes that regulate gene expression, enhance mitochondrial function, and improve DNA repair.
- FMD upregulates sirtuin activity, reducing oxidative damage and slowing aging.

AMPK Pathway Stimulation:

- AMPK (Adenosine Monophosphate-Activated Protein Kinase) is a metabolic master switch that enhances fat burning, increases insulin sensitivity, and promotes mitochondrial biogenesis.
- FMD triggers AMPK activation, improving energy efficiency and reducing metabolic disease risk.

Autophagy & Cellular Cleanup:

- FMD induces autophagy, a process where cells break down damaged organelles and misfolded proteins, reducing inflammation and neurodegenerative risk.
- This natural detoxification process lowers the burden of senescent (non-functioning) cells that contribute to aging and disease.

Reduced Inflammation & Immune System Rejuvenation:

- Short-term fasting lowers inflammatory cytokines, reducing systemic inflammation that contributes to chronic diseases.
- FMD has been shown to rejuvenate immune cells, increasing the production of new white blood cells and supporting immune system function.

Metabolic & Weight Loss Benefits:

- By maintaining a fasting-like state, FMD promotes fat loss while preserving lean muscle mass.
- It enhances ketone production, stabilizes blood sugar, and improves insulin sensitivity—key factors in preventing metabolic disorders like diabetes.

Key Benefits of the Fasting-Mimicking Diet:

- Promote Longevity: Increases lifespan and delays aging-related decline.
- Supports Fat Loss & Metabolic Health: Enhances fat burning, reduces insulin resistance, and improves lipid profiles.
- Boosts Brain Function: Reduces neuroinflammation, supports neurogenesis, and may protect against Alzheimer's and Parkinson's.
- Enhances Cellular Repair & Detoxification: Activates autophagy and DNA repair mechanisms.
- Strengthens the Immune System: Encourages immune cell regeneration and anti-inflammatory responses.
- Resets the Body for Optimal Function: A natural metabolic reset that supports hormonal balance and gut health.

How to Implement FMD Safely:

1. Choose a Five-Day Cycle: Repeat every 1-3 months, depending on health goals.
2. Follow a Low-Calorie, Plant-Based Diet: Prioritize whole foods, nuts, seeds, vegetables, and healthy fats.
3. Hydration is Key: Drink plenty of water, herbal teas, and electrolyte-rich beverages.
4. Minimize Heavy Exercise: Light movement (yoga, walking) is recommended to prevent excessive fatigue.
5. Reintroduce Food Gradually: After completing FMD, transition back to regular eating with whole, nutrient-dense foods.

By incorporating FMD into a long-term health strategy, individuals can harness the powerful benefits of fasting without the stress of complete food deprivation, promoting longevity, metabolic health, and cellular rejuvenation.

3.2.2. Nutrient-Dense Eating: Quality Over Quantity

Focusing on nutrient density ensures your body receives essential vitamins, minerals, and antioxidants with minimal empty calories. Staples of a nutrient-dense diet include:

Leafy Greens and Cruciferous Vegetables: Spinach, kale, broccoli, and Brussels sprouts are rich in vitamins and phytonutrients.

Seafood: Salmon, sardines, and oysters deliver omega-3s, zinc, and other vital nutrients.

Legumes and Seeds: Lentils, black beans, chia seeds, and pumpkin seeds provide protein, fiber, and essential minerals.

Whole Grains: Quinoa, barley, and farro are excellent sources of complex carbohydrates and fiber.

3.2.3. The Role of Nutraceuticals

<u>The Role of Nutraceuticals: Do We Really Need Supplements?</u>

In the modern era of health and wellness, the use of dietary supplements—often referred to as nutraceuticals—has skyrocketed. While these products promise numerous health benefits, ranging from improved immunity to enhanced cognitive function, the question remains: Do we truly need them? Furthermore, with a largely unregulated industry, how can consumers ensure they are purchasing safe, effective, and high-quality products?

The Lack of Regulation in the Supplement Industry

Unlike pharmaceuticals, which undergo rigorous testing and FDA approval before reaching consumers, most dietary supplements are not strictly regulated. In the United States, the Dietary Supplement Health and Education Act (DSHEA) of 1994 classifies supplements as a food category rather than drugs, allowing them to bypass many of the stringent safety and efficacy tests required for prescription medications. This lack of oversight leads to several concerns:

- Efficacy Issues: Many supplements on the market contain inadequate amounts of active ingredients, leading to minimal or no health benefits.
- Purity and Contamination: Without strict regulation, some supplements may contain contaminants, heavy metals, or even undisclosed pharmaceutical drugs.
- Misleading Claims: Manufacturers are not required to provide scientific proof for efficacy claims, leading to deceptive marketing and false promises.

Given these concerns, it is essential for consumers to rely on third-party tested products to ensure quality, safety, and effectiveness.

The Importance of Third-Party Testing

Because regulatory oversight is minimal, third-party testing is one of the most reliable ways to verify supplement quality. Reputable brands voluntarily subject their products to independent laboratory analysis to confirm:

- The presence of the ingredients listed on the label in the correct dosages

- The absence of harmful contaminants such as heavy metals, pesticides, and microbes
- The product's bioavailability and ability to be absorbed by the body

Third-party testing organizations, such as NSF International, USP (United States Pharmacopeia), ConsumerLab, and Informed Choice, provide certification that can help consumers distinguish high-quality products from inferior ones.

Recommended Dosing by Integrative and Functional Medicine Providers

Unlike conventional medicine, which often focuses on treating symptoms, integrative and functional medicine providers take a more personalized, preventative approach to health. They assess an individual's unique biochemical needs and recommend nutraceuticals tailored to their health concerns.

Key principles of dosing include:

1. Personalized Nutrition: Supplements should be chosen based on lab testing, symptoms, and lifestyle factors.
2. Evidence-Based Recommendations: Dosing should align with clinical research and best practices in functional medicine.
3. Bioavailability Considerations: Certain forms of nutrients (e.g., methylated B vitamins, liposomal vitamin C) offer superior absorption and effectiveness.

The Birth of Alphaceuticals: A Mission for High-Quality, Regulated Supplements

Recognizing the deficiencies in the supplement industry, Dr. Catherine founded Alphaceuticals, a company dedicated to producing highly regulated, premium-grade nutraceuticals.

Dr. Catherine's mission is simple: to bridge the gap between science-backed nutrition and consumer trust by ensuring that every product meets the highest standards for purity, potency, and efficacy.

What Sets Alphaceuticals Apart?

- Regulated Formulations: Every product is designed based on scientific evidence and manufactured under strict Good Manufacturing Practices (GMP).
- Partnerships with Third-Party Regulators: All supplements undergo independent testing for purity and quality.
- Clinically Effective Doses: Unlike many over-the-counter brands, Alphaceuticals ensures that dosages are in line with research-backed recommendations.
- Transparency & Traceability: Full disclosure of sourcing and manufacturing processes provides consumers with confidence in every purchase.

Buyer Beware: The Risks of Purchasing Supplements from Unverified Sources

With the rise of e-commerce, counterfeit and substandard supplements are rampant on online marketplaces. Purchasing from unauthorized sellers poses significant risks:

1. Contaminated Products: Some supplements may contain harmful ingredients, including fillers, additives, or toxins.
2. Expired or Degraded Ingredients: Without proper storage and handling, products may lose potency over time.
3. Fake Supplements: Certain brands are counterfeited and sold at lower prices with inactive or harmful substances.

How to Protect Yourself:

- Purchase only from trusted retailers or the brand's official website.
- Look for third-party certification logos on the packaging.
- Verify the manufacturer's GMP compliance and quality control practices.

Conclusion: Making Informed Choices for Optimal Health

Nutraceuticals can play a crucial role in optimizing health, filling nutritional gaps, and supporting disease prevention when used correctly. However, due to the lack of regulation in the supplement industry, it is vital to choose high-quality, third-party tested products from reputable sources. With brands like Alphaceuticals, consumers can finally access premium, science-backed formulations that offer both safety and efficacy.

By making informed choices, individuals can harness the true power of nutraceuticals while avoiding the pitfalls of an unregulated industry. Always consult a knowledgeable healthcare provider before starting any new supplement regimen to ensure it aligns with your unique health needs.

Consult an integrative and functional medicine practitioner to customize your supplementation regimen based on your health profile and goals.

3.3. Avoiding Longevity Saboteurs

What's Stealing Your Years?

While adopting longevity-enhancing habits is crucial, it's equally important to recognize and eliminate the hidden saboteurs that accelerate aging, increase disease risk, and sabotage metabolic health. The modern diet and lifestyle are rife with these culprits—some obvious, others lurking in plain sight.

3.3.1. Refined Sugar: The Sweet Enemy

Excess sugar is one of the most insidious contributors to chronic disease and premature aging. It fuels systemic inflammation, disrupts insulin sensitivity, and accelerates aging through **glycation**, a process where sugar molecules bind to proteins and fats, forming advanced glycation end-products (AGEs).

These compounds stiffen arteries, damage collagen, and contribute to conditions like diabetes, Alzheimer's, and cardiovascular disease.

How to Reduce Sugar's Damage:

- Swap sugary drinks for herbal teas, sparkling water with lemon, or black coffee.
- Use natural sweeteners like stevia, monk fruit, or allulose instead of artificial options.

- Satisfy cravings with fresh fruit, dark chocolate (70% cacao or higher), or nuts to curb blood sugar spikes.

3.3.2. Vegetable and Seed Oils: The Hidden Villains

Industrial seed oils—like canola, soybean, corn, and sunflower oil—are highly processed, oxidize easily, and contain an overabundance of omega-6 fatty acids, which drive chronic inflammation. They're linked to metabolic dysfunction, heart disease, and even neurodegeneration. Despite their misleading "heart-healthy" label, these oils are anything but beneficial.

Better Fat Choices:

- Extra Virgin Olive Oil – Rich in antioxidants and ideal for low-heat cooking or dressings.
- Avocado Oil – A stable option for high-heat cooking.
- Coconut Oil & Ghee – Excellent for sautéing and baking, with metabolism-boosting properties.

3.3.3. Processed Foods: The Silent Metabolic Wreckers

Highly processed foods—loaded with preservatives, artificial additives, and refined grains—strip away essential nutrients while flooding the body with chemicals that disrupt gut health and trigger inflammation. They're often engineered to be addictive, leading to overeating and metabolic dysfunction.

How to Reduce Processed Foods:

- Cook at home using whole, unprocessed ingredients.
- Prioritize single-ingredient foods (e.g., eggs, vegetables, meat, nuts).
- Read labels and avoid anything with a long list of unrecognizable ingredients.

3.3.4. Chronic Stress: The Silent Killer

Stress isn't just mental—it has profound physiological effects that accelerate aging. Chronic stress floods the body with cortisol, leading to high blood sugar, inflammation, and mitochondrial dysfunction. Over time, this increases the risk of cardiovascular disease, insulin resistance, and neurodegeneration.

How to Manage Stress Effectively:

- Practice deep breathing, meditation, or mindfulness daily.
- Engage in movement-based stress relief like yoga, tai chi, or nature walks.
- Prioritize quality sleep to regulate cortisol and promote recovery.

3.3.5. Sedentary Lifestyle: The Modern-Day Plague

Sitting is the new smoking—prolonged inactivity slows metabolism, weakens muscles, and contributes to insulin resistance. Regular movement is essential to maintaining muscle mass, cognitive function, and metabolic health.

How to Combat a Sedentary Lifestyle:

- Take movement breaks every 30–60 minutes (walk, stretch, or do squats).
- Incorporate daily low-intensity movement (walking, gardening, or standing desks).
- Engage in strength training to preserve muscle mass and prevent frailty.

Key Takeaway

Longevity isn't just about what you add to your life, it's also about what you remove. Cutting out refined sugars, inflammatory seed oils, ultra-processed foods, chronic stress, and excessive sitting can dramatically improve your metabolic health, brain function, and overall lifespan.

3.4. Lessons from Longevity Hotspots

The Secrets of the World's Healthiest People:

Across the globe, certain regions, often called *Blue Zones* or longevity hotspots, boast populations that not only live longer but thrive into their later years with vitality.

From the Mediterranean coast to the highlands of Central America and the islands of Japan, these communities share key lifestyle traits that foster exceptional longevity.

1. Mediterranean Longevity: The Art of Eating and Living Well

- Dietary Staples: Fresh vegetables, fruits, whole grains, legumes, olive oil, fish, and moderate wine consumption.

- Cultural Factors: Meals are a social affair, often enjoyed leisurely with family and friends. This sense of connection reduces stress and fosters emotional well-being.
- Movement: Daily activity is woven into life—whether it's walking, gardening, or light manual labor.
- Key Takeaway: Prioritizing whole, plant-based foods, healthy fats, and a communal dining culture can significantly improve longevity and overall well-being.

2. Okinawa, Japan: The Land of the Ageless

- Dietary Staples: Sweet potatoes (historically the main staple), tofu, seaweed, green tea, and an abundance of colorful vegetables.
- Mindset & Lifestyle: The Okinawans embrace *ikigai*—a strong sense of purpose—which has been linked to lower rates of stress and better mental health. They also practice *hara hachi bu*, eating until they are 80% full to prevent overeating.
- Physical Activity: Daily low-intensity movement, such as gardening, martial arts, and traditional dance, keeps them agile well into their later years.
- Key Takeaway: A plant-forward diet, portion control, and living with purpose create a foundation for longevity.

3. Nicoya Peninsula, Costa Rica: A Tropical Formula for Longevity

- Dietary Staples: Corn tortillas, black beans, squash, and tropical fruits, with a modest intake of protein (mostly from fish and eggs).

- Lifestyle & Community: Strong intergenerational family ties, deep spirituality, and daily physical labor contribute to well-being.
- Water Quality: The local water is naturally high in calcium and magnesium, which may contribute to lower rates of heart disease and stronger bones.
- Key Takeaway: Simple, nutrient-dense foods, close family bonds, and an active outdoor lifestyle foster long lives.

4. Ikaria, Greece: The Island Where People Forget to Die

- Dietary Staples: A variation of the Mediterranean diet, featuring wild greens, beans, potatoes, goat's milk, herbal teas, and small amounts of fish and meat.
- Relaxed Lifestyle: Afternoon naps and a low-stress attitude help maintain cardiovascular health.
- Community & Purpose: A strong sense of belonging, social cohesion, and engagement in community activities promote mental and emotional resilience.
- Key Takeaway: Stress reduction, strong social bonds, and a diet rich in antioxidants contribute to remarkable longevity.

5. Loma Linda, California: A Unique Blue Zone in the U.S.

- Dietary Staples: Many members of this Seventh-day Adventist community follow a vegetarian diet rich in nuts, legumes, and whole grains, with an emphasis on plant-based eating.

- Faith & Spirituality: A strong sense of faith and community support fosters emotional well-being and stress-resilience.
- Lifestyle Habits: Regular exercise, avoiding smoking and alcohol, and observing a Sabbath day of rest contribute to overall health.
- Key Takeaway: A plant-based diet, faith-based stress management, and community engagement enhance longevity.

Universal Longevity Lessons from Around the Globe

Despite geographic and cultural differences, these regions share common longevity-enhancing principles:

1. Plant-Based, Whole Foods Diet – Minimal processed foods, an abundance of vegetables, legumes, and healthy fats.
2. Strong Social Connections – Community bonds and family ties are essential for emotional resilience and lower stress levels.
3. Daily Natural Movement – Walking, gardening, and physical labor keep people active without structured workouts.
4. Stress Reduction & Purpose – Whether through faith, *ikigai*, or relaxed living, these cultures prioritize mental well-being.
5. Moderation in Eating – Portion control, fasting, or mindful eating practices help prevent overconsumption.

By incorporating these principles, we can adapt longevity-enhancing habits into modern life—wherever we live.

3.5. Putting It All Together

The path to longevity is paved with thoughtful choices. Start today by:

1. Fill half your plate with colorful vegetables.
2. Experimenting with a 12-hour overnight fast.
3. Swapping sugary snacks for nutrient-dense alternatives like nuts and seeds.
4. Upgrading your cooking oils to olive or avocado oil.
5. Incorporating anti-inflammatory spices like turmeric and ginger into your meals.
6. Avoid and mitigate environmental toxins.
7. Consulting a healthcare professional to tailor your supplements.

By adopting these strategies, you're not just adding years to your life, you're adding life to your years. Every meal becomes an opportunity to invest in a healthier, more vibrant future.

CHAPTER 4
THE GUT MICROBIOME

Your Body's Hidden Superpower

Welcome to the wild world of your gut, bustling metropolis of trillions of microscopic residents working tirelessly to keep you alive, energized, and happy. The gut isn't just about digestion; it's about unlocking one of the greatest secrets to longevity and optimal health. Meet your gut microbiome, the ultimate behind-the-scenes health hero!

4.1. Gut Check: What Is the Microbiome?

Your gut microbiome is a vast community of bacteria, viruses, fungi, and other microorganisms primarily residing in your intestines. With over 100 trillion microbes calling your gut home, they outnumber your human cells 10 to 1. Even more staggering, the genetic material of these microbes surpasses your human DNA by a ratio of 150 to 1. It's not an exaggeration to say that we're as microbial as we are human. This symbiotic partnership plays an essential role in nearly every facet of your health, making it critical to nurture this microscopic ecosystem.

4.2. Why Your Gut Is the CEO of Your Health

Think of your gut as the command center of your body. While its most well-known role is digestion, the gut also impacts immune function, mental health, metabolism, and even the rate at which you age. Here's how:

- Immune System Guardian: Approximately 70% of your immune system resides in the gut. The gut microbiome trains immune cells to recognize harmful invaders while preventing overreactions that could lead to autoimmune conditions or allergies.

- Mood Regulator: Known as the second brain, your gut produces up to 90% of serotonin, the "feel-good" hormone. A healthy gut supports a balanced mood and better emotional resilience.
- Metabolism Overseer: Your gut microbes break down food, extract nutrients, and influence fat storage. A balanced microbiome ensures efficient digestion and metabolic harmony.
- Inflammation Control: Beneficial gut bacteria lower inflammation, which is implicated in almost every chronic disease, from arthritis to Alzheimer's.
- Nutrient Factory: Certain gut bacteria synthesize essential nutrients like vitamin K and B vitamins, acting as a biochemical factory within your body.

4.3. The Gut-Brain Axis: Your Second Brain

The gut and brain are in constant dialogue via the gut-brain axis, a bi-directional communication network involving the central nervous system, the enteric nervous system, and the microbiome. This connection explains how gut health directly impacts mental clarity, mood, and cognitive performance.

- Neurotransmitter Production: Gut bacteria produce serotonin, dopamine, and GABA—key players in mood regulation, memory, and focus.
- Vagus Nerve Communication: The vagus nerve acts as a direct hotline between the gut and brain. Activities like deep breathing, yoga, and meditation enhance vagal tone, supporting this vital communication.

- Dysbiosis and Cognitive Decline: Imbalances in the gut microbiome (dysbiosis) have been linked to anxiety, depression, and even neurodegenerative conditions like Parkinson's and Alzheimer's disease. A healthy gut fosters a sharp, balanced mind.

4.4. Microbiome Diversity and Longevity: More Bugs, More Benefits

A diverse microbiome is a hallmark of good health and longevity. Microbial diversity contributes to stronger immunity, better digestion, and a reduced risk of chronic illnesses.

- Diverse Gut, Longer Life: Studies show that a richer microbiome reduces inflammation, promotes immune balance, and supports healthy aging.
- Probiotics and Prebiotics: Probiotics are live beneficial bacteria found in foods like yogurt, kefir, and kimchi. Prebiotics, the fiber-rich foods that fuel these bacteria—include bananas, asparagus, garlic, and onions.
- Cutting-Edge Therapies: Fecal Microbiota Transplantation (FMT) is emerging as a powerful tool to restore gut health, particularly for conditions like Clostridium difficile infections. Though unconventional, it highlights the transformative potential of microbiome therapy.
- Molecular hydrogen plays a pivotal role in supporting gut health by acting as a powerful antioxidant and anti-inflammatory agent. It can help balance the microbiome by reducing oxidative stress, promoting the growth of beneficial bacteria, and inhibiting harmful microbes. Additionally, molecular hydrogen

may improve gut barrier integrity, reducing the risk of leaky gut and systemic inflammation. It also influences gut-mitochondria interactions, enhancing energy production at the cellular level. By supporting a balanced microbiome, molecular hydrogen contributes to overall health and longevity.

4.5. Gut-Immune Connection: The Body's Defense System

The gut's connection to the immune system cannot be overstated. The gut-associated lymphoid tissue (GALT) acts as the body's frontline defense, identifying and neutralizing harmful pathogens.

- Leaky Gut and Chronic Disease: When the gut lining becomes overly permeable ("leaky gut"), toxins and bacteria enter the bloodstream, triggering systemic inflammation. This condition is linked to autoimmune diseases, metabolic syndrome, and other chronic conditions.
- Repairing Gut Integrity: Foods and nutrients that heal the gut lining include bone broth (rich in collagen and amino acids), L-glutamine (a key fuel source for gut cells), and probiotics like Lactobacillus and Bifidobacterium strains.

4.6. The Gut's Electrical Potential and Energy Production

Your gut isn't just a digestive organ; it plays a role in bioenergetics. The gut lining maintains an electrical potential, creating a charge gradient essential for nutrient absorption and communication between cells.

- Gut-Mitochondria Link: The microbiome influences mitochondrial function, the powerhouse of your cells. Healthy gut bacteria produce short-chain fatty acids (SCFAs) like butyrate, which fuel mitochondria and enhance energy production.
- Electrochemical Signals: These signals ensure efficient nutrient transport and facilitate communication between the gut and other organs, amplifying your body's energy output.

4.7. Foods and Nutrients for a Healthy Gut

Fuel your gut with these microbiome-friendly superstars:

- Fermented Foods: Yogurt, sauerkraut, kimchi, and miso provide live probiotics to populate your gut with beneficial bacteria.
- High-Fiber Foods: lentils, beans, and fruits like apples and berries serve as prebiotics, nourishing beneficial microbes.
- Polyphenol-Rich Foods: Green tea, dark chocolate, and brightly colored fruits combat oxidative stress and support gut health.
- Collagen-Rich Foods: Bone broth and collagen supplements help repair the gut lining.
- Omega-3 Fatty Acids: Found in fatty fish, chia seeds, and flaxseeds, these fats reduce inflammation in the gut.

4.8. Strategies for Optimal Gut Health

Nurture your microbiome with these actionable strategies:

1. Eat a Diverse Diet: Incorporate a variety of whole, minimally processed foods to support microbial diversity.
2. Prioritize Fermented Foods: Add probiotics to your diet with kefir, kombucha, and fermented vegetables.
3. Stay Hydrated: Adequate water intake supports digestion and nutrient absorption.
4. Limit Processed Foods: Reduce sugar and artificial additives, which disrupt microbial balance.
5. Manage Stress: Chronic stress weakens the gut lining and disrupts the microbiome. Incorporate stress-relief practices like meditation or deep breathing.
6. Get Regular Sleep: Sleep disturbances negatively impact gut health. Aim for 7-9 hours per night.

4.9. Gut Health and Personalized Strategies

Every gut is unique, and tailoring your approach ensures the best results:

- Microbiome Testing: Tools like stool analysis and microbiome sequencing can reveal the specific needs of your gut.
- Targeted Interventions: Based on testing, you might increase fiber, introduce specific probiotics, or eliminate certain foods.
- Functional Medicine Approach: Work with professionals who are certified and trained in functional and integrative medicine to create a personalized gut health plan that aligns with your overall wellness goals.

Final Thoughts: Trust Your Gut (Literally)

Your gut microbiome is one of the most powerful tools for a longer, healthier, and happier life. By feeding and nurturing the trillions of microorganisms in your gut, you're investing in vibrant health, enhanced mood, sharper cognition, and sustained energy. Remember, you're not just what you eat, you're what your microbes do with what you eat. Treat your gut kindly, and it will reward you in ways you never imagined.

Here's to a thriving gut and a thriving you!

CHAPTER 5
MOVEMENT AS MEDICINE

The Role of Physical Activity in Longevity

Movement is the ultimate life hack. Not just the kind that involves rearranging your furniture or pacing while on a call, but intentional, purposeful activity that has the power to extend your healthspan and lifespan. Exercise is more than a calorie burn or a way to fit into your favorite jeans; it's a daily prescription for vitality, impacting your body on a cellular level and acting as a shield against chronic disease. In this chapter, we'll dive deep into the science of movement as medicine, examining how it transforms your body and why it's essential for a longer, healthier life.

Mitochondria: The Powerhouses of Life and Longevity

Mitochondria, the microscopic organelles nestled in your cells, are much more than energy factories. These structures convert nutrients into adenosine triphosphate (ATP), the energy currency that powers nearly every process in your body. Your brain firing on all cylinders? Thank you for your mitochondria. Your heart beating effortlessly? Credit goes to them. These organelles are central to health, aging, and vitality.

Your body contains approximately 37.2 trillion cells, with each cell housing between 100 and 10,000 mitochondria, depending on its energy demands. High-energy organs like the brain, heart, and muscles are mitochondrial hubs. Collectively, these organelles produce around 10 billion ATP molecules per day per cell, amounting to roughly your entire body weight in ATP daily. It's no exaggeration to say that energy is life, and mitochondria are the engines.

Beyond ATP production, mitochondria play several critical roles. They regulate apoptosis, or programmed cell death, which prevents the buildup of damaged cells that could lead to cancer or degenerative diseases. They maintain calcium homeostasis, essential for muscle contractions, nerve signaling, and blood clotting. Additionally, mitochondria manage reactive oxygen species (ROS), balancing their role as cellular signaling molecules and their potential to cause oxidative stress when overproduced. Even hormone synthesis relies on mitochondria, as they produce key steroid hormones that influence stress responses and reproductive health.

However, as we age, mitochondrial efficiency declines. Damaged mitochondria produce less energy and more oxidative stress, a phenomenon linked to age-related conditions like neurodegenerative diseases, cardiovascular disorders, and metabolic dysfunctions. Protecting and enhancing mitochondrial function is, therefore, pivotal for longevity.

Exercise is one of the most effective ways to boost mitochondrial health. Aerobic activities like running or cycling promote mitochondrial biogenesis, increasing their number and efficiency. Resistance training preserves muscle strength and stimulates mitochondrial adaptation, while high-intensity interval training (HIIT) maximizes energy efficiency and mitochondrial growth. Pairing movement with nutritional strategies—like a ketogenic diet or intermittent fasting—activates pathways like AMPK and PGC-1α, enhancing mitochondrial repair and energy production.

Supplements such as Coenzyme Q10 and alpha-lipoic acid also support mitochondrial health.

A low-carb diet, particularly one rich in healthy fats and moderate protein, has profound effects on mitochondrial function, the powerhouse of our cells. By reducing carbohydrate intake, the body shifts from relying on glucose for energy to primarily burning fat, a process that produces ketones. Ketones serve as a highly efficient fuel source, generating more ATP per molecule compared to glucose while producing fewer reactive oxygen species (ROS), which can reduce oxidative stress and cellular damage. This metabolic shift enhances mitochondrial biogenesis—the creation of new mitochondria—leading to improved energy production, resilience against age-related decline, and better metabolic flexibility. Additionally, low-carb and ketogenic diets activate pathways like AMPK and sirtuins, which support mitochondrial repair, longevity, and overall cellular health. By optimizing mitochondrial function, a low-carb lifestyle may contribute to increased energy levels, cognitive clarity, and even longevity.

Practices like cold exposure, sauna use, stress management, and quality sleep further optimize these cellular engines, ensuring you have the vitality to live a full, active life.

5.1. Exercise and Cellular Aging

Physical activity does more than make you feel good in the moment; it impacts your cells in profound ways. Telomeres, the protective caps on your DNA, shorten with age, leading to cellular aging.

Exercise, however, helps maintain telomere length, effectively slowing the aging process. Studies show that even modest activities, like brisk walking for 30 minutes five days a week, can have significant anti-aging effects. This daily investment pays dividends, keeping your cells healthier for longer.

Exercise also improves mitochondrial function, enabling your cells to produce energy efficiently and repair damage. Regular movement reduces systemic inflammation, balances hormones, and optimizes glucose metabolism, all of which contribute to cellular longevity. By making exercise a non-negotiable part of your routine, you're giving your cells the best chance to thrive.

5.2. Cardiovascular Exercise: Heart and Soul of Longevity

Cardiovascular exercise, or cardio, is the gold standard for heart health, brain function, and metabolic resilience. Whether it's running, swimming, cycling, or even an impromptu dance-off with your kids, regular cardio improves circulation, lowers blood pressure, and helps regulate cholesterol levels by increasing HDL (the "good" cholesterol) and reducing LDL (the "bad" cholesterol). But the benefits extend far beyond your heart. Studies show that consistent cardio can reduce the risk of dementia by up to 30% by increasing blood flow to the brain, enhancing neuroplasticity, and reducing inflammation. It also serves as a powerful stress reliever, triggering the release of endorphins—your body's natural mood elevators.

Cardiometabolic Health: More Than Just a Strong Heart

Beyond the immediate cardiovascular benefits, cardio plays a key role in overall cardiometabolic health by improving insulin sensitivity and supporting mitochondrial efficiency.

Mitochondria—the energy-producing powerhouses of cells—thrive with regular aerobic exercise, increasing ATP production and reducing oxidative stress. This directly lowers the risk of metabolic disorders like type 2 diabetes, obesity, and insulin resistance.

A Deep Dive into Lipoproteins: The Hidden Players in Heart Disease

Cardio helps optimize key lipoproteins that determine cardiovascular risk beyond just standard cholesterol numbers:

Lipoprotein(a) [Lp(a)]: This genetically influenced lipoprotein is a strong predictor of heart disease, independent of LDL or HDL levels. High Lp(a) can promote arterial plaque formation and clotting, increasing heart attack and stroke risk. Regular cardio, along with dietary and lifestyle interventions, may help reduce its impact.

Apolipoprotein A1 (ApoA1): The main component of HDL, ApoA1 is responsible for reverse cholesterol transport, removing excess cholesterol from the bloodstream and arteries. Higher ApoA1 levels are associated with a lower risk of heart disease.

Apolipoprotein B (ApoB): Found in LDL and VLDL particles, ApoB is a more accurate marker of cardiovascular risk than standard LDL measurements. It represents the total number of atherogenic (plaque-forming) particles in circulation, meaning lower ApoB levels are better for heart health.

Making Cardio a Sustainable Habit:

To make cardio an effortless part of your routine, start small and focus on consistency. Interval walking—alternating between fast and slow paces—can be just as effective as running for cardiovascular benefits. Incorporate movement into daily life by walking while on calls, using stairs instead of elevators, or even vacuuming with extra vigor. The key is finding activities you enjoy, making cardio feel less like a chore and more like an investment in your heart, brain, and longevity.

5.3. Strength Training: Your Armor Against Aging

Muscle mass naturally declines with age, a process called sarcopenia. By the time you reach 30, you may start losing 3-8% of your muscle mass with each passing decade. Strength training counters this decline, preserving muscle and bone density while boosting metabolism. It's also essential for maintaining balance and preventing falls as you age.

Begin with simple bodyweight exercises like squats, lunges, and push-ups. As you progress, incorporate resistance bands or weights to challenge your muscles.

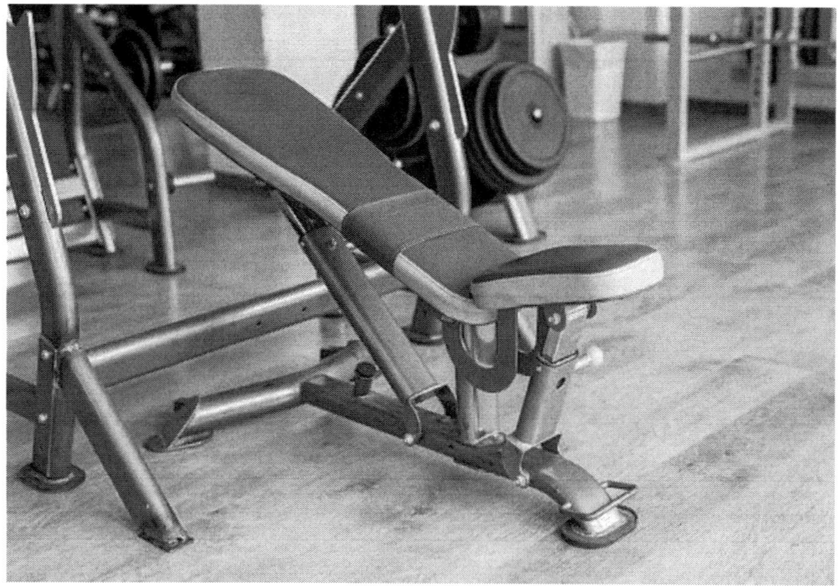

further. Schedule two strength-training sessions per week and gradually increase intensity. Strength training is more than just building muscle; it's about building resilience and safeguarding your independence as you are aging.

5.4. Flexibility and Mobility: The Unsung Heroes

Flexibility and mobility are often overlooked in fitness routines, but they're critical for injury prevention and smooth movement. Stretching improves muscle elasticity and joint health, while mobility exercises enhance your range of motion, making daily activities easier and safer. Practices like yoga or Pilates not only increase flexibility but also improve balance and core strength, further reducing injury risks.

Dedicate 5-10 minutes each day to stretching. Incorporate dynamic stretches, like leg swings and arm circles, before workouts and use static stretches afterward to cool down. Flexibility and mobility may not get as much attention as cardio or strength training, but they are the glue that holds your fitness together.

5.5. Exercise as Medicine for Disease Prevention

Movement is one of the most powerful tools for preventing chronic diseases. Aerobic exercise strengthens your heart, reduces blood pressure, and improves cholesterol profiles, lowering your risk of cardiovascular disease. Resistance training improves insulin sensitivity, making it a potent weapon against type 2 diabetes. Physical activity also reduces systemic inflammation, a key driver of many chronic conditions, including certain cancers.

The cumulative effect of regular exercise is profound: better immune function, improved metabolic health, and reduced inflammation. By moving regularly, you're not just adding years to your life; you're adding life to your years.

5.6. Recovery and Resilience: Rest Like a Pro

Recovery is where magic happens. While exercise stresses your body, recovery allows it to adapt, repair, and grow stronger. Active recovery, like a gentle walk or restorative yoga, promotes blood flow and reduces muscle stiffness. Sleep is another cornerstone of recovery, as it facilitates mitochondrial repair and reduces cortisol levels.

Incorporate foam rolling or stretching into your routine to release muscle tension. Schedule rest days and prioritize quality sleep to ensure your body can rebuild and recharge. Recovery isn't a break from progress; it's an essential part of it.

5.7. In Summary: Movement is Medicine

Exercise is not a chore; it's a celebration of what your body can do. From energizing mitochondria to maintaining cellular health, protecting your heart, and sharpening your mind, movement is the ultimate prescription for longevity. By making physical activity a consistent and enjoyable part of your life, you're not just extending your years; you're ensuring they're filled with vitality, purpose, and joy. So go ahead—dance, stretch, lift, and run like your life depends on it. Because, in many ways, it does.

CHAPTER 6
OPTIMIZING SLEEP FOR LONGEVITY

6.1. The Science of Sleep

Sleep is the unsung hero of health and longevity—a nightly opportunity to recharge, repair, and reset. Yet, in our fast-paced, screen-filled world, it often takes a backseat to late-night Netflix binges and endless to-do lists. The truth is, neglecting sleep can sabotage your health and accelerate aging. Let's dive into the science of sleep, discovering what happens when you're dreaming (or not) and how to make the most of your nightly rest.

6.1.1. Understanding Sleep Stages

Sleep isn't just one long, uninterrupted state. It's a symphony of stages, each playing a vital role in your physical and mental health:

- **Light Sleep (Stages 1 and 2)**: The gateway to deeper sleep, light sleep is where your body begins to relax, and your heart rate and breathing slow down. It makes up about 50% of your sleep cycle.
- **Deep Sleep (Stage 3)**: This is the restorative stage where your body focuses on repair. Growth hormone is released, tissues are rebuilt, and your immune system is strengthened.
- **REM Sleep**: The stage where dreams come alive. REM sleep is crucial for cognitive functions like memory consolidation, learning, and emotional regulation. It accounts for 20-25% of your sleep cycle.

Each stage serves a unique purpose, and cycling through them 4-6 times per night is essential for rejuvenation.

6.1.2. The Glymphatic System: Brain Detox at Night

While you sleep, your brain goes into cleanup mode. The glymphatic system—a waste-removal process—flushes out toxins like beta-amyloid plaques, which are associated with Alzheimer's disease. This nightly detox reduces the risk of neurodegenerative diseases and keeps your brain sharp. Missing out on quality sleep is like skipping garbage day; waste builds up, and your brain pays the price.

6.1.3. Sleep and Hormones: The Body's Balancing Act

Sleep regulates key hormones that affect everything from metabolism to mood:

- Cortisol: Known as the stress hormone, cortisol levels should naturally dip at night and rise in the morning. Poor sleep disrupts this cycle, leading to fatigue and weight gain.
- Melatonin: The sleep hormone, melatonin is triggered by darkness and helps regulate your circadian rhythm. Light exposure at night can suppress melatonin, throwing off your sleep-wake cycle.
- Growth Hormone: Released during deep sleep, growth hormone is essential for tissue repair, muscle growth, and fat metabolism.

Skipping sleep doesn't just make you tired; it throws your entire hormonal orchestra out of tune.

6.2. Circadian Rhythms: Your Body's Internal Clock

Your circadian rhythm is the natural 24-hour cycle that governs your sleep-wake patterns, body temperature, and even digestion. Aligning your lifestyle with this internal clock is a cornerstone of health and longevity.

6.2.1. Melatonin and Cortisol: The Yin and Yang of Sleep

Melatonin and cortisol work in tandem to regulate sleep and wakefulness. Melatonin rises as darkness falls, signaling your body it's time to wind down. Meanwhile, cortisol peaks in the morning, giving you the energy to start your day. Disruptions to this cycle—like staying up late or waking inconsistently—can lead to fatigue, brain fog, and increased disease risk.

6.2.2. Light Exposure: The Key to Healthy Rhythms

Natural light exposure in the morning helps anchor your circadian rhythm by boosting cortisol production and suppressing melatonin. In contrast, blue light from screens at night interferes with melatonin release, making it harder to fall asleep. Aim for 10-15 minutes of sunlight exposure upon waking and minimize screen time at least an hour before bed.

6.2.3. Chrononutrition: Eating by the Clock

When you eat matters as much as what you eat. Eating late at night can disrupt your circadian rhythm, leading to poor sleep and weight gain. Align your meals with your body's natural cycles by:

- Eating a nutrient-dense breakfast within an hour of waking.

- Consuming your largest meal during daylight hours.
- Avoiding heavy meals or snacks at least three hours before bedtime.

6.3. Common Sleep Disorders and Their Impact

Sleep disorders can wreak havoc on health and longevity, but understanding and addressing them is the first step toward better sleep.

Insomnia

Difficulty falling or staying asleep, insomnia affects millions and is often fueled by stress, anxiety, or poor sleep hygiene. Chronic insomnia can lead to fatigue, mood disorders, and even cardiovascular issues.

Sleep Apnea

This condition, characterized by interrupted breathing during sleep, increases the risk of heart disease, stroke, and diabetes. Symptoms include loud snoring, gasping for air, and excessive daytime sleepiness.

Restless Leg Syndrome (RLS)

RLS causes uncomfortable sensations in the legs, leading to an irresistible urge to move them. It disrupts sleep quality and can contribute to fatigue and irritability.

Integrative Approaches to Sleep Disorders

- Cognitive-Behavioral Therapy for Insomnia (CBT-I): A proven method for retraining your brain to sleep better.

- Herbal Remedies: Supplements like valerian root, magnesium, and chamomile can support relaxation.
- Lifestyle Changes: Regular exercise, stress management, and a consistent sleep schedule are foundational.
- For treatment of sleep apnea: a combination of weight loss management, positional therapy, PAP therapy, oral appliance or Inspire (hypoglossal nerve stimulation device).

6.4. Creating the Ideal Sleep Environment

Your bedroom should be a sanctuary for sleep. A well-designed sleep environment minimizes disruptions and promotes deep, restorative rest.

Optimize Your Environment:

- Lighting: Use blackout curtains and dim lighting in the evening to support melatonin production.
- Temperature: Keep your bedroom cool, ideally between 60-67°F (15-19°C), to promote sleep onset.
- Bedding: Invest in a comfortable mattress and breathable, high-quality linens.

Pre-Sleep Routines

Wind-down routines signal to your body that it's time for sleep. Consider relaxing activities like reading, meditating, or gentle stretching. Avoid stimulating activities like intense exercise or emotional conversations right before bed.

Technology and Sleep

Technology is a double-edged sword. While blue light from screens suppresses melatonin, excessive EMF exposure may interfere with sleep quality. Minimize screen time before bed and consider keeping devices out of the bedroom entirely. If you must use screens, invest in blue light-blocking glasses or enable night mode on your devices.

6.5. Solutions for Better Sleep

- Stick to a Schedule: Go to bed and wake up at the same time every day, even on weekends.
- Prioritize Morning Sunlight: Exposure to natural light in the morning resets your circadian rhythm.
- Limit Caffeine and Alcohol: Both can interfere with deep sleep and should be avoided in the hours leading up to bedtime.
- Do not eat right before bed: this can disrupt sleep by interfering with your body's natural nighttime processes. Late-night meals can spike blood sugar and insulin levels, making it harder to fall asleep and stay in restorative deep sleep. Additionally, digestion competes with the body's repair mechanisms, reducing sleep quality and potentially leading to discomfort or acid reflux. To optimize sleep, aim to finish eating at least 2-3 hours before bedtime.
- Practice Relaxation Techniques: Deep breathing, progressive muscle relaxation, or mindfulness meditation can help calm your mind and prepare you for sleep.
- Visualization can be a powerful tool for improving sleep by calming the mind and reducing stress. By imagining peaceful, soothing scenarios—like walking

along a beach or lying under a starry sky—you engage your brain's relaxation response, slowing your heart rate and easing tension. This mental imagery shifts your focus away from racing thoughts, helping you drift off into restful sleep.

In Summary: Sleep Your Way to Longevity

Sleep is the foundation of health, influencing everything from brain function to immune resilience. By understanding the science of sleep, aligning your habits with your circadian rhythm, and creating an optimal sleep environment, you can unlock the restorative power of sleep to enhance your longevity and vitality. Remember, every hour of quality sleep is an investment in a longer, healthier, and more energetic life. So, turn off the lights, silence your phone, and let sleep work its magic.

CHAPTER 7
MANAGING STRESS AND BUILDING RESILIENCE

The Impact of Chronic Stress on Aging

Stress is like that annoying houseguest who overstays their welcome. A little stress now and then can motivate you, but chronic stress? That's the guest who eats all your snacks, leaves dirty dishes everywhere, and sets fire to your health. Chronic stress accelerates aging, wreaks havoc on your body, and sets the stage for chronic diseases. The good news? You don't have to let it take over—understanding its impact and mastering stress-busting strategies is your secret weapon for vitality.

7.1. Stress and Cellular Aging

Imagine your DNA wearing a pair of shoes with shoelaces; the telomeres are the plastic tips at the ends of those laces. Chronic stress chews on those tips, making your cellular shoelaces fray faster. Elevated cortisol levels accelerate telomere shortening, leading to premature aging and increased risk of diseases like cancer and heart disease. Worse yet, stress also brings along its toxic pals—oxidative stress and inflammation—to wreak even more cellular havoc. But fear not, by shuffling stress out the door, you can slow down the wear and tear on your cellular shoelaces.

Cortisol: The Double-Edged Sword

Cortisol is your body's natural Red Bull—a quick boost when you need it most. But when the boost doesn't stop, it turns into a slow-dripping poison. Chronic cortisol elevation messes with your metabolism, weakens your immune defenses, and even shrinks the hippocampus (your brain's memory command center). Think of cortisol like fire, it's great in a fireplace but disastrous when it's out of control.

The Inflammatory Cascade

Stress sets off an inflammatory domino effect in your body. Imagine your immune system in a constant state of DEFCON 1. Over time, this hyper-vigilance damages tissues, increases oxidative stress, and contributes to diseases like Alzheimer's, arthritis, and depression. Chronic inflammation turns your body's defense system into its worst enemy, but dialing down stress can calm the storm and bring your body back to balance.

7.2. Mind-Body Practices: Tools for Stress Reduction

The brain and body are like an old married couple—always talking to each other, whether they're in sync or not. Mind-body practices help smooth out that relationship, reducing stress and promoting resilience. Here's how you can take charge of your mental and physical harmony.

Meditation and Mindfulness

Meditation isn't about chanting on a mountaintop (though that's cool too). It's about quieting the mental chatter that keeps you stuck in a loop of "what-ifs" and "should-haves." Regular meditation has been shown to lower cortisol levels, reduce anxiety, and improve focus. Even 10 minutes a day can work wonders. Add some mindfulness to the mix, like savoring your morning coffee instead of gulping it down, and you'll find stress has less room to breathe.

Breathwork: The Science of Relaxation and Deep Release

Breathing isn't just for survival; it's a superpower hiding in plain sight. Controlled breathwork can shift your nervous system from fight-or-flight to full-body Zen in mere minutes. Techniques like box breathing (inhale for 4, hold for 4, exhale for 4) can lower your heart rate faster than watching a cat video on the internet. Meanwhile, somatic breathwork dives even deeper, using conscious, rhythmic breathing to unlock stored tension, release emotional blockages, and reset your body's stress response.

Why does it work? Breathwork activates your parasympathetic nervous system (a.k.a. your chill mode), helping to regulate cortisol, lower blood pressure, and restore balance. Somatic techniques take it a step further, guiding you through patterns of deep, connected breathing that can induce a profound state of relaxation, heightened awareness, and even emotional breakthroughs.

Bonus: It's free, portable, and always available. Your breath is the one tool that never runs out of battery, doesn't need Wi-Fi, and works every time—if you know how to use it.

Praying

Praying, studying, and meditating on the Bible deepen your spiritual connection and foster a stronger, more vibrant faith.

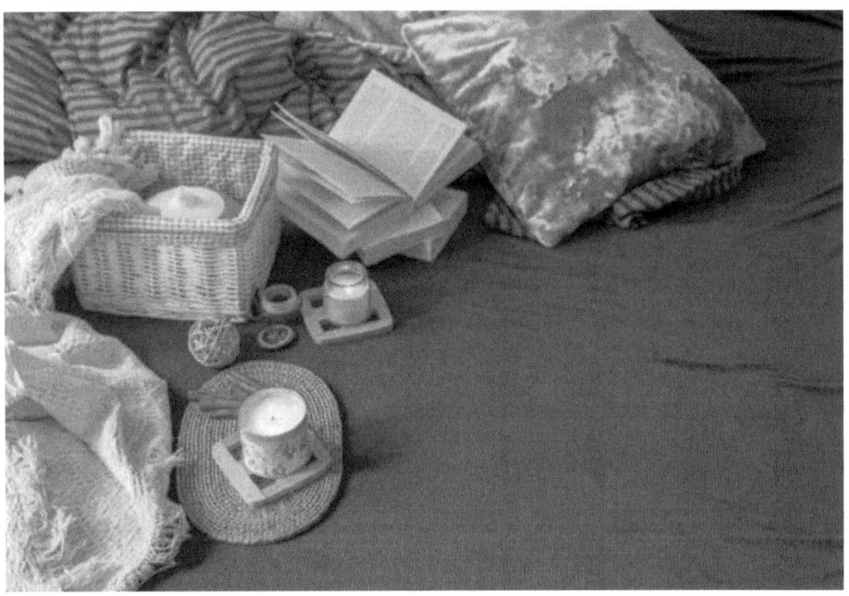

Integrating Mind-Body Practices

Formal practices like yoga and tai chi are stress-busting Swiss Army knives. They combine movement, breath, and mindfulness for a triple-threat approach to relaxation. But even informal practices—like taking a mindful walk or pausing to stretch—can help you reset. Experiment with what works for you and make it a habit. Your future self will thank you.

7.3. Hormesis and Resilience: Stress That Strengthens

Not all stress is the villain. Small, controlled stressors—a concept called hormesis—can make you stronger. Think of it as training your body to handle life's curveballs.

The Role of Hormesis

Hormesis is like sending your body to boot camp. Controlled stressors like exercise, fasting, or temperature changes activate repair mechanisms, improve mitochondrial function, and build resilience. Your body loves a good challenge—in moderation.

Cold Exposure and Sauna Therapy

Cold showers and ice baths might sound torturous, but they're resilience-building gold. Cold exposure activates brown fat, boosts metabolism, and releases norepinephrine (your brain's natural pep talk). On the flip side, saunas heat things up, improving cardiovascular health and stimulating heat shock proteins that repair damaged cells. Together, they're like a spa day for your resilience.

Psychological Resilience

Building mental toughness is like strengthening a muscle. Cognitive reframing helps you see challenges as opportunities. Stress inoculation trains you to handle adversity by gradually increasing your exposure to manageable stressors. Pair that with a growth mindset and practices like journaling or gratitude, and you'll become the Rocky Balboa of stress management.

7.4. Community and Relationships: The Buffer Against Stress

Strong relationships are like bubble wrap for your soul. They cushion you against life's bumps and bruises, providing emotional support and a sense of belonging.

The Role of Social Connections

Science backs it up: People with strong social networks have lower cortisol levels, better immune function, and longer lives. Meaningful connections release oxytocin, the hormone that makes you feel warm and fuzzy inside while countering the effects of stress. In short, friends are nature's anti-stress prescription.

Loneliness and Mortality

Loneliness isn't just sad; it's deadly. It's as bad for your health as smoking a pack of cigarettes a day. Lonely individuals have higher inflammation and a greater risk of chronic diseases. Building connections isn't just nice, it's essential for survival.

Building and Maintaining Relationships

Cultivating relationships takes effort, but the payoff is huge. Listen more, talk less, and show empathy. Share activities, celebrate wins, and support each other during tough times. Join clubs, volunteer, or simply call a friend. Your social circle is your safety net, so keep it strong.

7.5. Strategies for Managing Stress

Stress management isn't about eliminating stress altogether (good luck with that). It's about building a toolkit to handle it effectively. Here are a few staples:

- Physical Activity: Move your body. Whether it's a dance party in your living room or a brisk walk, exercise is a proven stress buster.
- Sleep Hygiene: Sleep is your body's reset button. Stick to a schedule, make your bedroom a sanctuary, and avoid scrolling your phone in bed.
- Nutrition: Fuel your body with stress-fighting foods like salmon (omega-3s), spinach (magnesium), and dark chocolate (yes, chocolate). Avoid caffeine overload and sugary crashes.
- Time Management: Prioritize tasks, delegate when possible, and don't be afraid to say no. Overcommitment is a fast track to burnout.
- Therapeutic Practices: Therapy isn't just for crisis mode. Cognitive-behavioral techniques help you reframe stress and develop coping strategies.

7.6. Creating a Resilient Lifestyle

Building resilience is like assembling a life toolkit. It's not just about avoiding stress but thriving despite it. Incorporate stress-relieving practices, strengthen your social connections, and embrace challenges as opportunities to grow. With the right mindset and habits, you can transform stress from an enemy into a teacher.

Remember, stress is like a bad haircut: unavoidable, but manageable with the right tools. With humor, resilience, and a little self-care, you've got this.

CHAPTER 8 DETOXIFICATION AND ENVIRONMENTAL HEALTH

Nurturing Longevity through Detoxification and Environmental Wellness

Welcome to your body's personal cleanup crew headquarters! Every day, you're exposed to a parade of environmental toxins, from air pollution to household chemicals, and your body's natural detoxification system works overtime to keep you safe. But just like a hardworking office team, these systems need support to thrive. This chapter dives into the art and science of detoxification and environmental health, showing you how to lend a helping hand to your body's detox heroes and create a toxin-free sanctuary for optimal longevity.

8.1. Detoxification and Environmental Health

Detoxification is your body's way of saying, "Out with the bad, in with the good." It's the natural process of removing harmful substances, ensuring your internal systems run smoothly. Meanwhile, environmental health focuses on reducing the external factors that threaten your wellness. Together, they form the ultimate power duo for promoting longevity and vitality. By understanding toxins and their effects, and taking action to support your body's detox pathways, you're setting the stage for a healthier, happier you.

Understanding Toxins and Their Impact

From the air you breathe to the food you eat, toxins are everywhere. Common culprits include air pollutants like smog and industrial chemicals, water contaminants such as heavy metals and pesticides, and food additives like artificial sweeteners and preservatives. Household items like cleaning products, air fresheners, and plastics also contribute to your toxin load. These everyday exposures can disrupt endocrine function, damage cells, and accelerate aging. Over time, toxins accumulate in the body, overburdening detox pathways and increasing the risk of chronic illnesses such as cancer, diabetes, and autoimmune disorders.

The Body's Natural Detoxification Processes

Your body is equipped with a sophisticated detox system involving the liver, kidneys, lungs, skin, and lymphatic system. The liver acts as the star of this show, processing toxins through its two-phase detoxification process. In Phase I, toxins are chemically altered into intermediate substances, which are often highly reactive. Phase II neutralizes these intermediates, converting them into water-soluble compounds for elimination through bile or urine. The kidneys filter blood to expel waste through urine, the lungs expel volatile toxins through exhalation, and the skin eliminates waste via sweat. Meanwhile, the lymphatic system transports waste and immune cells, ensuring the body's drainage system works efficiently.

To keep these systems functioning optimally, it's essential to support them with nutrient-dense foods, regular movement, and hydration.

8.2. Detoxification Strategies for Longevity

8.2.1. Dietary Support

A diet rich in cruciferous vegetables (broccoli, kale, Brussels sprouts), antioxidant-packed fruits (berries, oranges, and cherries), and high-fiber foods (beans, flaxseeds, and whole grains) fuels the body's detox pathways. These foods support liver enzymes, bind toxins in the gut, and combat oxidative stress. Adding healthy fats like avocado and walnuts further supports cell membrane integrity, aiding toxin transport and excretion.

Hydration is another cornerstone of detoxification. Adequate water flushes toxins through the kidneys and supports lymphatic flow. Herbal teas like dandelion, nettle, and green tea provide added detox benefits.

8.2.2. Fasting and Autophagy

Intermittent fasting stimulates autophagy, a natural process where your body breaks down and recycles damaged cells. This cellular "deep cleaning" helps eliminate accumulated toxins and reduces oxidative damage. Short-term juice cleanses can complement fasting, offering a concentrated nutrient boost while resting the digestive system.

8.2.3. Lifestyle Enhancements

Incorporating practices like yoga, walking, and regular exercise promotes circulation, supports lymphatic flow, and enhances oxygen delivery to cells, aiding the detox process. Sweat-inducing activities like saunas and cardio workouts encourage the release of toxins through the skin.

8.2.4. Functional Medicine and Personalized Detoxification

Functional medicine takes detoxification to a personalized level by addressing unique health imbalances and environmental exposures. Testing for heavy metals, persistent organic pollutants (POPs), or genetic variants influencing detox enzyme activity allows for customized strategies. For instance, individuals with sluggish Phase II liver pathways may benefit from targeted supplementation, such as glutathione precursors or sulfur-rich foods like garlic and onions.

8.2.5. Creating an Environment for Longevity

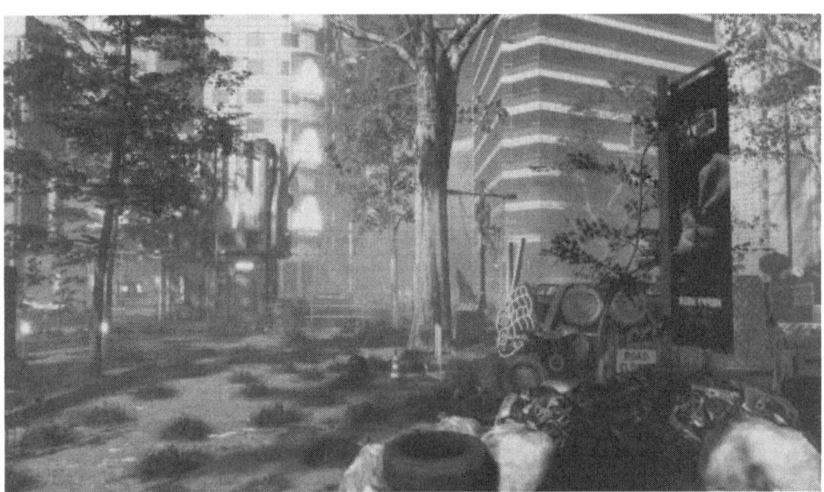

Your external environment plays a significant role in reducing your toxin burden. Opting for organic produce to minimize pesticide exposure, and filter your water to remove contaminants like chlorine, lead, and microplastics. Use non-toxic cleaning products and avoid synthetic fragrances found in air fresheners and candles. Plants like peace lilies, spider plants, and bamboo palms not only beautify your space but also improve indoor air quality by filtering volatile organic compounds (VOCs).

Decluttering your home and reducing stress-inducing visual noise can also promote mental clarity and overall well-being, indirectly supporting detoxification.

Mold Toxicity and Chronic Inflammatory Response Syndrome (CIRS):

Mold toxicity is a serious and often overlooked health concern resulting from exposure to toxic mold species commonly found in water-damaged buildings. These molds release mycotoxins, harmful compounds that can trigger widespread inflammation, immune dysfunction, and neurological impairment when inhaled, ingested, or absorbed through the skin. Symptoms of mold toxicity can range from chronic fatigue and respiratory issues to cognitive decline and persistent inflammation, often mimicking other chronic illnesses. If left unaddressed, mold toxicity can evolve into a complex, multi-system condition known as Chronic Inflammatory Response Syndrome (CIRS).

<u>Understanding Chronic Inflammatory Response Syndrome (CIRS)</u>

CIRS is a systemic inflammatory illness triggered by prolonged exposure to biotoxins. Unlike an acute immune response, where the body effectively neutralizes and eliminates harmful substances, individuals with CIRS experience a dysregulated immune system that fails to shut off the inflammatory cascade. This leads to chronic, unresolved inflammation affecting multiple organs and systems, including the brain, muscles, joints, gastrointestinal tract, and respiratory system.

One of the biggest challenges with CIRS is its broad spectrum of symptoms, which often overlap with conditions like Lyme disease, chronic fatigue syndrome, fibromyalgia, and autoimmune disorders. Without proper diagnosis, many patients struggle for years with unexplained symptoms, unaware that their environment may be the root cause of their suffering.

Causes and Risk Factors for CIRS

While mold exposure in water-damaged buildings is the most well-known trigger for CIRS, other biotoxins can also cause this condition, including:

- Mycotoxins from mold (common in homes, schools, and workplaces with water damage)
- Harmful algae blooms (cyanobacteria toxins) from contaminated water sources
- Tick-borne illnesses, such as Lyme disease, which can introduce persistent biotoxins
- Certain spider and insect bites that introduce neurotoxic compounds into the body

Who is at Risk?

Some individuals are more susceptible to CIRS than others. Key risk factors include:

- Genetic Predisposition: Certain genetic variants make it difficult for some people to clear biotoxins efficiently.
- Prolonged Exposure: Living or working in a mold-contaminated environment for extended periods increases risk.

- Weakened Immune System: Individuals with autoimmune conditions or chronic infections are more vulnerable.
- Compromised Detoxification Pathways: Poor liver function, gut health imbalances, and sluggish lymphatic drainage can contribute to toxin buildup.

Symptoms of Mold Toxicity and CIRS

CIRS is a multi-system illness, meaning symptoms can manifest in various parts of the body. Common symptoms include:

Neurological and Cognitive Symptoms:

- Brain fog, memory loss, and difficulty concentrating
- Headaches and dizziness
- Mood swings, anxiety, and depression

Respiratory and Sinus Issues:

- Shortness of breath and chest tightness
- Chronic sinus congestion and recurrent infections

Muscle and Joint Symptoms:

- Unexplained muscle aches and joint pain
- Weakness and persistent fatigue

Metabolic and Hormonal Disruptions:

- Unexplained weight gain or loss
- Temperature dysregulation and night sweats

Gastrointestinal Problems:

- Bloating, diarrhea, nausea, and abdominal pain
- Food sensitivities and difficulty digesting fats

Many patients experience a combination of these symptoms, making it difficult to pinpoint the root cause without specialized testing.

Diagnosis and Testing for CIRS

Diagnosing CIRS requires a comprehensive evaluation that includes medical history, symptom assessment, and specialized lab testing. Some of the most reliable diagnostic tools include:

Visual Contrast Sensitivity (VCS) Test: This non-invasive eye test measures the ability to detect subtle visual patterns, which is often impaired in individuals with CIRS.

Genetic Testing: Specific HLA-DR gene variants can indicate genetic susceptibility to biotoxin-related illnesses.

Laboratory Biomarkers: A range of blood tests can reveal:

- Inflammatory markers (e.g., C-reactive protein, TGF-beta 1)
- Immune dysfunction indicators (e.g., low MSH, high VEGF)
- Mycotoxin levels (detected via urine mycotoxin testing)

Treatment Approaches for Mold Toxicity and CIRS

Successful treatment of mold toxicity and CIRS requires a multi-faceted approach that includes eliminating exposure, detoxifying the body, and restoring immune function.

1. Identifying and Eliminating Mold Exposure

- Mold Remediation: If mold is found in your home or workplace, professional remediation is essential.
- Air Purification: HEPA filters and activated carbon purifiers can help reduce airborne mold spores.
- Environmental Testing: Regular mold testing ensures your living space remains safe.

2. Detoxification and Biotoxin Removal

- Binders: Cholestyramine, activated charcoal, and bentonite clay help trap and remove toxins.
- Liver Support: Glutathione, milk thistle, and N-acetylcysteine (NAC) enhance detox pathways.
- Sweating & Lymphatic Support: Infrared saunas, dry brushing, and rebounding can aid detox.

3. Supporting the Immune System & Reducing Inflammation

- Low-inflammatory diet: Focus on whole, nutrient-dense foods and avoid processed foods, sugar, and inflammatory oils.
- Supplements: Omega-3 fatty acids, vitamin D, and curcumin help modulate the immune response.
- Hormone Balancing: Many CIRS patients experience hormonal disruptions that require targeted support.

4. Managing Symptoms & Restoring Health

- Gut Health: Probiotics, prebiotics, and digestive enzymes support a balanced microbiome.
- Neurological Support: Cognitive therapy, nootropic supplements, and brain retraining techniques can improve mental clarity.
- Stress Reduction: Meditation, breathwork, and adaptogenic herbs help regulate cortisol levels.

Preventive Measures: Protecting Your Health from Mold and Biotoxins

Preventing mold toxicity and CIRS starts with creating a toxin-free environment and maintaining a resilient immune system. Key strategies include:

Mold Prevention:

- Regularly inspect water leaks, condensation, and mold growth in your home.
- Use dehumidifiers in damp areas to keep humidity levels below 50%.
- Ensure proper ventilation in moisture-prone areas, such as kitchens and bathrooms.

Strengthen Detox Pathways:

- Drink plenty of filtered water to flush the toxins.
- Eat anti-inflammatory foods rich in antioxidants and fiber.
- Engage in regular movement to promote lymphatic drainage and circulation.

Dr. Olusegun Oseni: A Leading Mold and CIRS Expert in Texas

At Alpha Care Wellness Center, we are proud to have Dr. Olusegun Oseni, one of the leading mold and CIRS specialists in Texas. His expertise in diagnosing and treating biotoxin-related illnesses has helped countless patients regain their health after struggling with unexplained symptoms for years.

Conclusion: Take Control of Your Health Today

Mold toxicity and CIRS are complex but treatable conditions that require a comprehensive approach to diagnosis, treatment, and prevention. If you suspect mold exposure is affecting your health, don't wait—early intervention is key to recover.

At Alpha Care Wellness Center, we specialize in providing cutting-edge, holistic treatments for mold-related illnesses. Contact us today to schedule a consultation and start your journey toward healing.

8.2.6. Phase 3 Detoxification

The Final Step in Cellular Cleansing

Detoxification is a multi-step process that enables the body to eliminate harmful substances, including toxins from the environment, metabolic waste, and byproducts of cellular metabolism. While Phase 1 and Phase 2 detoxification focus on breaking down and transforming toxins into water-soluble compounds, Phase 3 detoxification is the critical final step—ensuring these toxins are efficiently transported out of the body.

Phase 3 detox primarily involves cellular transporters, such as multidrug resistance proteins (MRPs) and P-glycoproteins, which actively move toxins and metabolic waste from cells into bile, urine, sweat, and feces for excretion. This phase occurs in key detox organs like the liver, kidneys, intestines, and lymphatic system. Without proper Phase 3 detox, toxins can re-circulate in the body, leading to oxidative stress, inflammation, and chronic health issues.

Optimizing Phase 3 Detoxification for Longevity and Health

For effective detoxification, supporting Phase 3 is just as crucial as the earlier phases, ensuring toxins don't get stuck in the body. Several key factors influence this phase:

- Bile Flow and Gut Health – The liver packages toxins into bile, which is then eliminated through the intestines. Supporting bile flow with bitter foods (e.g., dandelion greens, artichokes) and fiber-rich foods prevents toxin reabsorption.
- Hydration and Kidney Function – Drinking adequate water and consuming electrolytes (like potassium and magnesium) ensures efficient toxin removal through urine.
- Sweating and Lymphatic Support – Infrared saunas, exercise, and dry brushing help mobilize toxins out of fat cells and into the lymphatic system for elimination.
- Binder Support – Activated charcoal, bentonite clay, and modified citrus pectin can help trap and eliminate toxins, reducing their chances of being reabsorbed in the gut.

Why Phase 3 Detox Matters for Longevity:

Inefficient Phase 3 detoxification leads to a buildup of metabolic waste, heavy metals, and environmental toxins that contribute to chronic inflammation, mitochondrial dysfunction, and accelerated aging. Supporting this phase ensures that detoxification is not just a temporary cleanse but an ongoing process that enhances energy, brain function, and overall longevity. By integrating movement, hydration, gut health support, and natural detox enhancers, you can keep your body's detox pathways working efficiently for a lifetime of optimal health.

8.3. The Alpha Cellular Restoration Program

In a world where chronic illness is the norm and aging seem like an unstoppable decline; the pursuit of lasting health has never been more critical. Despite the influx of wellness trends—superfoods, biohacking, and anti-aging protocols—one fundamental aspect is often ignored: the body's ability to detoxify at a cellular level.

We live in a sea of toxins. From the air we breathe to the food we eat and the water we drink, pollutants infiltrate every aspect of our daily lives. Industrial chemicals, pesticides, heavy metals, and endocrine disruptors silently accumulate in our bodies, wreaking havoc on our metabolism, hormones, and overall vitality. Even personal care products and household items—innocuous as they seem—are laced with hidden toxins that seep into our skin and bloodstream.

Yet the real danger isn't just exposure, it's accumulation. These toxins don't simply exit the body unnoticed; they embed themselves in tissues, cells, and fat stores, leading to a cascade of biological dysfunction. Fatigue, brain fog, inflammation, hormonal imbalances, and unexplained weight gain are the body's distress signals—early warnings that detoxification pathways are overloaded. When left unchecked, toxic buildup sets the stage for autoimmune conditions, cardiovascular disease, neurodegeneration, and even cancer.

The Alpha Cellular Restoration Program: A Science-Backed Detox for Optimal Health

The good news? Detoxification isn't a myth or a fleeting wellness trend—it's a biological necessity. The body is equipped with powerful detoxification systems, primarily the liver, kidneys, gut, and lymphatic system. However, in today's toxic landscape, these organs often struggle to keep pace, requiring targeted support to function at peak efficiency.

This is where the Alpha Cellular Restoration Program comes in—a scientifically designed, comprehensive approach to restoring balance, enhancing detoxification pathways, and revitalizing cellular health. Unlike quick-fix cleanses, this program doesn't just eliminate toxins; it optimizes mitochondrial energy, supports liver function, and resets metabolic efficiency for long-term resilience.

By integrating strategic nutrition, cutting-edge supplementation, and detox-supportive lifestyle practices, the Alpha Cellular Restoration Program systematically removes harmful substances, reduces inflammation, and revitalizes your body from the inside out. The result? Increased energy, sharper cognition, improved digestion, and a newfound sense of vitality.

The Science of Detoxification: How Toxins Disrupt Metabolism

Every day, we encounter thousands of synthetic chemicals which didn't exist a century ago. These substances interfere with cellular function, impair energy production, and disrupt hormonal balance. Stress, poor diet, and sleep deprivation further compound the problem, slowing down detox pathways and allowing toxins to recirculate rather than be eliminated.

To truly optimize health, detoxification must be a daily, strategic process—not just an occasional cleanse. The Alpha Cellular Restoration Program works by:

- Activating Liver Detoxification – Enhancing Phase I & II detox pathways to neutralize and eliminate toxins.
- Balancing the Gut Microbiome – Preventing toxin reabsorption and improving digestion.
- Boosting Mitochondrial Energy – Ensuring detoxification is fueled by optimal cellular energy.
- Enhancing Antioxidant Protection – Neutralizing free radicals to prevent oxidative damage and inflammation.
- Supporting Lymphatic Drainage – Stimulating the body's natural waste-removal system.

<u>The Alpha Cellular Restoration Kit: Your Detox Powerhouse</u>

To optimize detoxification, targeted supplementation is essential. The Alpha Cellular Restoration Kit is a curated selection of nutraceuticals designed to fortify each stage of the detox process:

- Alpha ATP Energy – Supports mitochondrial function and fuels detoxification pathways with key nutrients like B vitamins, CoQ10, and alpha-lipoic acid.

- Alpha Detox Protein – Provides liver-supportive amino acids, fiber, and polyphenols to enhance toxin elimination and digestive health.
- Alpha LipoCare – A powerhouse blend of milk thistle, dandelion root, and bile-stimulating compounds to enhance liver detoxification and hormone balance.

Each component works synergistically to ensure toxins are not only mobilized but efficiently processed and eliminated, preventing toxin recirculation and metabolic stagnation.

Beyond Detox: A Blueprint for Lifelong Vitality

Detoxification is not a one-time event—it is an ongoing strategy for longevity. By maintaining detox-supportive habits, you can sustain the benefits long after completing the program. This includes:

- Eating nutrient-dense, organic foods that fuel liver detox pathways.
- Prioritizing hydration to facilitate toxin elimination.
- Engaging in movement and sweating (via exercise or sauna) to enhance lymphatic flow.
- Optimizing sleep to support the glymphatic system, your brain's natural detox network.
- Reducing exposure to environmental toxins by choosing clean beauty, household, and food products.

The Path to a Healthier, Longer Life Starts Today

True health is not about quick fixes—it's about sustainable, science-backed strategies that support the body's natural ability to detoxify, heal, and regenerate. By integrating the Alpha Cellular Restoration Program into your lifestyle, you can reclaim your energy, clarity, and resilience—ensuring a future where your body functions at its peak for years to come.

Detoxification is not a trend; it is a necessity for thriving in the modern world. Now is the time to take control of your health, optimize your cellular function, and unlock a new level of vitality. The journey to lifelong wellness begins now.

8.4. Emerging Therapies and Practices

The landscape of detoxification therapies is continually evolving, offering cutting-edge tools to enhance your body's natural processes:

Saunas and Infrared Therapy

Sweating is one of the most effective ways to eliminate toxins, and saunas take it to the next level. Infrared saunas penetrate deeper into tissues, promoting detoxification at the cellular level while enhancing circulation and reducing inflammation. Regular use has been shown to support cardiovascular health and improve recovery from environmental toxin exposure.

Chelation Therapy

Chelation therapy involves the use of agents like EDTA to bind heavy metals and remove them from the body. While effective for specific toxic exposures, it should be conducted under professional supervision due to potential nutrient depletion. Alternatives like natural chelators, such as chlorella and cilantro, offer gentler options for heavy metal detox.

Molecular Hydrogen

Molecular hydrogen acts as a selective antioxidant, neutralizing harmful free radicals without disrupting beneficial signaling molecules. This emerging therapy supports cellular repair, reduces oxidative stress, and enhances mitochondrial function, making it a valuable addition to detox protocols.

High-Frequency Vibration Therapy

Using vibration platforms or devices, this therapy enhances lymphatic drainage, promoting the removal of waste products and improving circulation. It's particularly effective for those with sedentary lifestyles or conditions that limit physical activity.

Photo-biomodulation and Analog PEMF

Photo-biomodulation uses red and near-infrared light to boost mitochondrial energy production, supporting detoxification at a cellular level. Analog PEMF (Pulsed Electromagnetic Field Therapy) stimulates tissue repair and enhances detoxification by improving cellular communication and oxygen delivery.

8.5. Conclusion: Embracing Detoxification and Environmental Health

Detoxification isn't about quick fixes or drastic measures. It's about consistent, sustainable practices that support your body's natural processes and minimize toxic exposures. By making thoughtful changes to your diet, lifestyle, and environment, you can create a cleaner, healthier foundation for longevity. Emerging therapies offer exciting opportunities to enhance these efforts, blending ancient wisdom with modern innovation.

So, grab your water bottle, stock up on greens, and let's toast to a cleaner, brighter future—because your body deserves nothing less.

CHAPTER 9
THE HARMONY OF HORMONES

Your Body's Secret Longevity Orchestra

Hormones are your body's backstage pass to optimal health. These powerful messengers, produced by your endocrine glands, regulate everything from metabolism to mood, stress response, and even how you age. Picture hormones as the orchestra, peptides as the sheet music, and your body as the stage. When they're in tune, it's a symphony of vitality. When they're not? It's like an out-of-sync orchestra—offbeat, disjointed, and hard to ignore. Let's delve into the world of hormonal balance, how it shifts as we age, and how to keep the music playing beautifully.

9.1. The Aging Endocrine System: Changes That Keep Us on Our Toes

Aging doesn't just add gray hairs; it orchestrates a hormonal remix. The endocrine system, which includes glands like the pituitary, thyroid, and adrenal glands, shifts its hormone production. Estrogen, testosterone, growth hormone, and thyroid hormones—all face declines, creating ripple effects throughout the body.

As women age, estrogen—the hormone that supports bone density, cognitive function, and heart health—declines dramatically with menopause. This shift increases risks for osteoporosis, heart disease, and memory lapses. Men, on the other hand, experience a gradual decrease in testosterone starting in their 30s, which can lead to muscle loss, lower libido, and reduced energy. Growth hormone, your body's rejuvenator, also takes a hit with age. Reduced levels lead to decreased muscle mass, increased fat accumulation, and slower tissue repair. Meanwhile, a sluggish thyroid can result in fatigue, weight gain, and cognitive fog. Together, these shifts make managing hormones a cornerstone of longevity.

While acute cortisol is your best friend in emergencies, chronic stress keeps this "fight-or-flight" hormone elevated. Elevated cortisol wreaks havoc on metabolism, immune function, and brain health. This chronic overload accelerates aging by promoting inflammation and oxidative damage—two villains in the longevity saga.

9.2. Peptides: The Unsung Heroes of Longevity

Peptides—tiny but mighty—are short chains of amino acids that serve as the body's biochemical messengers. Think of them as text messages sent between cells, delivering precise instructions on how to repair, regenerate, and optimize biological functions. Unlike bulky proteins, peptides are streamlined and efficient, capable of stimulating everything from tissue repair and fat metabolism to brain function and immune support.

The best part? Science is now unlocking their potential for longevity, anti-aging, and disease prevention. Whether you're looking to boost mitochondrial function, support cognitive health, improve muscle mass, or reduce inflammation, peptides might just be the cheat code for living a longer, healthier life.

How Peptides Benefit Us: Supercharging the Body from Within

As we age, cellular processes slow down, hormones decline, and our body's ability to repair itself weakens. Peptides can step in and reactivate dormant functions, helping to:

- Regenerate tissues – Peptides can stimulate growth factors, improving skin elasticity, muscle recovery, and joint health.
- Enhance mitochondrial function – By optimizing energy production, peptides help increase vitality, endurance, and cognitive clarity.
- Boost the immune system – Some peptides regulate T-cell function, making the body more resilient to infections and diseases.
- Balance hormones – From improving insulin sensitivity to boosting growth hormone levels, peptides play a key role in metabolic health.
- Support brain function – Cognitive-enhancing peptides sharpen memory, focus, and mental agility—critical for longevity.

Peptides are not one-size-fits-all but rather target specific pathways to restore optimal function where it's needed most.

The Most Popular Peptides for Longevity

1. BPC-157: The Ultimate Repair Peptide

Nicknamed "The Wolverine Peptide", BPC-157 is a powerful healing agent derived from gastric juices. It accelerates tissue repair, reduces inflammation, and supports gut health. Athletes love it for muscle and joint recovery, but its benefits extend to healing leaky gut, improving brain function, and even protecting against organ damage.

- Best for: Injury recovery, gut health, inflammation control
- How it works: Increases blood flow and stimulates angiogenesis (new blood vessel formation)
- Fun fact: It has been shown to heal torn ligaments and reduce arthritis symptoms!

2. Epitalon: The Longevity Timekeeper

Epitalon is a pineal gland peptide that activates telomerase, an enzyme responsible for lengthening telomeres (the protective caps on your DNA). Shorter telomeres are a marker of aging, so by extending them, Epitalon is believed to slow aging, improve sleep, and boost cellular repair.

- Best for: Longevity, anti-aging, improved sleep
- How it works: Stimulates telomerase production to extend telomere length
- Fun fact: Russian scientists have studied Epitalon for decades as an anti-aging intervention!

3. Thymosin Alpha-1 (Tα1): The Immune Warrior

This peptide is a master regulator of the immune system, enhancing T-cell function and reducing chronic inflammation. It's particularly effective in fighting autoimmune diseases, infections, and even certain cancers.

- Best for: Immune support, inflammation control, disease prevention

- How it works: Enhances the production and function of T-cells (immune warriors)
- Fun fact: It's being researched as a potential COVID-19 treatment for immune modulation.

4. CJC-1295 & Ipamorelin: The Growth Hormone Duo

This dynamic peptide combo stimulates natural growth hormone release, leading to increased muscle mass, fat loss, improved sleep, and cellular repair. Unlike synthetic HGH, these peptides work by encouraging your body to produce its own growth hormone naturally, reducing the risk of side effects.

- Best for: Fat loss, muscle growth, recovery, deep sleep
- How it works: Stimulates the pituitary gland to release more natural growth hormone
- Fun fact: Many biohackers use this duo as a safer alternative to HGH therapy.

5. MOTS-c: The Mitochondrial Booster

MOTS-c is a mitochondrial-derived peptide that acts like a cellular energy optimizer. It improves insulin sensitivity, increases metabolism, and boosts endurance, making it a favorite for those looking to enhance longevity and combat age-related decline.

- Best for: Metabolic health, energy levels, endurance
- How it works: Regulates mitochondrial energy production and promotes fat metabolism

- Fun fact: Known as the "exercise mimetic," MOTS-c provides similar benefits to exercise without working out!

6. Cerebrolysin: The Brain Booster

Cerebrolysin is a neuropeptide cocktail that enhances brain function, memory, and neuroprotection. It is commonly used to treat neurodegenerative diseases like Alzheimer's, but it's also gaining traction as a cognitive enhancer for longevity seekers.

- Best for: Brain health, memory, neuroprotection
- How it works: Promotes neurogenesis (new brain cell growth) and prevents oxidative stress in the brain
- Fun fact: It was originally developed to improve stroke recovery and dementia symptoms.

How to Incorporate Peptides for Longevity

Peptides can be administered in different ways depending on their function:

- Injections – The most effective method for bioavailability. Common for growth hormone peptides and immune modulators.
- Oral Peptides – Some peptides, like BPC-157, can be taken in capsule form.
- Topical & Nasal Sprays – Certain peptides, like Melanotan II (for tanning) and Selank (for anxiety), can be absorbed through the skin or nasal passages.

Pro Tip: Not all peptides are created equal! Quality matters, so always source from reputable compounding pharmacies or specialized clinics.

The Future of Peptides in Longevity Science

The explosive growth in peptide research is reshaping the future of longevity medicine. Scientists are now exploring peptides that reverse aging at the cellular level, enhance cognitive performance, and even repair DNA damage. In the coming years, we can expect new peptide discoveries that may push the boundaries of human lifespan and healthspan even further.

Whether you're looking to boost muscle, sharpen cognition, improve metabolic health, or slow aging, peptides offer a cutting-edge, science-backed approach to optimizing human performance and longevity.

So, are peptides the future of longevity? The science says yes—just don't wait too long to jump on board!

9.3. Insulin Sensitivity: A Key to Metabolic Longevity

Insulin resistance isn't just a precursor to diabetes; it's a driver of accelerated aging. When cells stop responding effectively to insulin, the body produces more of it, creating a vicious cycle that promotes inflammation and oxidative stress. Over time, this can lead to chronic conditions like heart disease, Alzheimer's, and obesity.

Improving insulin sensitivity is crucial. Low-glycemic foods like leafy greens, whole grains, and healthy fats stabilize blood sugar levels, while resistance training and aerobic exercise increase glucose uptake into muscles. Supplements such as berberine, alpha-lipoic acid, and chromium offer additional support, helping the body maintain balanced insulin levels. Cultivating metabolic flexibility—the ability to switch seamlessly between burning carbs and fats—further enhances longevity by reducing metabolic strain.

9.4. Adrenal Health: The Stress Managers of the Body

Your adrenal glands, perched atop your kidneys, are the architects of your stress response. They produce cortisol and adrenaline, hormones essential for responding to immediate stressors. However, chronic stress can exhaust these glands, leading to adrenal fatigue. Symptoms include exhaustion, brain fog, and weakened immunity.

To support adrenal health, adaptogens like ashwagandha, rhodiola, and holy basil work wonders by regulating cortisol production and improving stress resilience. Regular meals with protein, healthy fats, and complex carbs help stabilize blood sugar, reducing unnecessary cortisol spikes. Mindfulness practices, such as yoga and meditation, offer additional stress management, promoting a sense of calm and balance.

9.5. Bioidentical Hormone Replacement Therapy (BHRT): The Science of Youthful Balance

Aging is inevitable, but hormonal decline doesn't have to be. Enter Bioidentical Hormone Replacement Therapy (BHRT)—a modern, personalized approach to restoring hormonal balance and optimizing health as we age. Unlike traditional Hormone Replacement Therapy (HRT), which often uses synthetic or animal-derived hormones, BHRT utilizes hormones that are chemically identical to those naturally produced by the body. This bioidentical precision allows for greater effectiveness, fewer side effects, and improved safety, making BHRT a game-changer in longevity medicine.

Why Hormonal Balance Matters for Longevity

Hormones orchestrate nearly every function in the body, from metabolism and energy production to cognitive function, muscle strength, and emotional well-being. As we age, levels of key hormones—such as estrogen, progesterone, testosterone, DHEA, thyroid hormones, and cortisol—begin to decline or become imbalanced, leading to a cascade of age-related symptoms, including:

- Fatigue and brain fog
- Weight gain and sluggish metabolism
- Mood swings, anxiety, and depression
- Decreased muscle mass and bone density
- Low libido and sexual dysfunction
- Hot flashes, night sweats, and sleep disturbances

BHRT provides a targeted, science-backed solution to address these imbalances, allowing both men and women to regain vitality, enhance longevity, and maintain optimal health well into later years.

<u>The Benefits of BHRT for Men and Women</u>

BHRT for Women: A Menopause & Perimenopause Lifeline

For women, hormonal fluctuations begin well before menopause—sometimes in their late 30s or early 40s—leading to symptoms of perimenopause, which can last years before full menopause sets in. BHRT helps to stabilize hormones, alleviating uncomfortable symptoms and protecting long-term health.

Key Benefits for Women:

- Menopause & Perimenopause Relief – Reduces hot flashes, night sweats, mood swings, and sleep disturbances
- Bone Health – Estrogen supports bone density, reducing the risk of osteoporosis
- Cognitive Function – Protects brain health, reducing the risk of Alzheimer's and cognitive decline
- Heart Health – Balances cholesterol levels and vascular function, decreasing cardiovascular risks
- Sexual Wellness – Restores libido, vaginal lubrication, and overall sexual function

Estrogen & Progesterone: The Dynamic Duo

- Estrogen (Estradiol, Estriol, Estrone): Maintains bone density, skin elasticity, brain function, and heart health.
- Progesterone: Acts as a natural calm-inducing hormone, helping with anxiety, mood stabilization, and sleep.

BHRT for Men: Revitalizing Testosterone & Vitality

While men don't experience menopause in the same way, they gradually lose testosterone over time—a process known as andropause. This leads to a decline in energy, strength, cognitive sharpness, and sexual health. BHRT helps men restore testosterone levels naturally, improving:

- Muscle Mass & Strength – Increases lean muscle retention and improves fat metabolism
- Energy & Mood – Boosts motivation, confidence, and mental clarity
- Heart Health – Testosterone plays a role in blood vessel function and cholesterol regulation
- Libido & Sexual Function – Enhances desire, erectile function, and overall performance

Testosterone: The Hormone of Masculinity & Longevity

Low testosterone is linked to obesity, diabetes, cardiovascular disease, and cognitive decline. BHRT can reverse these risks, helping men maintain their strength, vitality, and mental acuity as they age.

Personalized Hormone Therapy: One Size Does Not Fit All

Unlike traditional hormone therapy, BHRT is not a one-size-fits-all approach. It is customized based on individual needs and lab testing.

Step 1: Comprehensive Hormone Testing

- Saliva, urine, or blood testing to assess current hormone levels.
- Evaluates estrogen, progesterone, testosterone, thyroid function, cortisol, and DHEA levels.

Step 2: Customized BHRT Protocol

- Bioidentical hormones are tailored to the exact dose and delivery method that suits you best.

- Delivery methods include creams, gels, injections, sublingual drops, or pellet implants.

Step 3: Ongoing Monitoring & Adjustments

- Regular follow-ups ensure hormones stay balanced and side effects are minimized.
- Adjustments are made based on symptom improvements and lab results.

Myths & Misconceptions About BHRT

Myth #1: "All hormone therapy increases cancer risk." Fact: Unlike synthetic HRT, bioidentical hormones do not carry the same risks. Proper monitoring ensures safe usage.

Myth #2: "Hormone therapy is only for menopause." Fact: Men and women of all ages can benefit from hormone balancing—whether due to perimenopause, andropause, or early hormonal decline.

Myth #3: "You just need testosterone or estrogen." Fact: Optimal hormone health involves a balance between estrogen, progesterone, testosterone, thyroid hormones, and cortisol. BHRT is about harmony, not excess.

The Role of BHRT in Longevity & Disease Prevention

Beyond symptom relief, BHRT is an anti-aging tool with long-term protective effects:

- Protects Against Heart Disease – Regulates cholesterol, blood pressure, and arterial function.
- Preserves Brain Health – Reduces risk of Alzheimer's and cognitive decline.

- Prevents Muscle Loss – Maintains lean muscle, strength, and metabolism.
- Reduces Osteoporosis Risk – Strengthens bone density and prevents fractures.

As part of a comprehensive longevity strategy, BHRT helps restore youthfulness, energy, and healthspan, making it an essential pillar in anti-aging medicine.

Is BHRT Right for You?

If you're experiencing chronic fatigue, weight gain, brain fog, mood swings, or low libido, your hormones might be out of sync. A simple test can provide insight into your hormone levels and whether BHRT could restore your vitality and extend your healthspan.

Take the Next Step: Consult a hormone specialist or longevity doctor to see if BHRT is the missing piece in your anti-aging and wellness journey.

Conclusion: BHRT – The Modern Approach to Aging Gracefully

Aging doesn't have to mean declining energy, sluggish metabolism, or reduced quality of life. With personalized bioidentical hormone therapy, you can maintain optimal health, vitality, and longevity. Whether you're a man seeking to restore testosterone or a woman looking to balance estrogen and progesterone, BHRT offers a safe, effective way to age powerfully and gracefully.

Why accept hormonal decline as inevitable? BHRT lets you take control, optimize your health, and live your best life—at any age.

9.6. Emerging Therapies and Innovations

Peptide therapies are at the forefront of longevity science, offering targeted solutions for aging pathways. These include muscle repair, immune modulation, and even cognitive enhancement. Functional medicine approaches, which evaluate genetics, lifestyle, and environmental factors, help tailor interventions to individual needs. Nutritional strategies like incorporating phytoestrogens (found in soy) and omega-3 fatty acids further support hormonal balance. Meanwhile, artificial intelligence is revolutionizing personalized medicine, analyzing vast datasets to optimize peptide and hormonal therapies.

9.7. Conclusion: The Symphony of Longevity

Your hormones and peptides are the maestros of your body's orchestra, orchestrating every note of your health. Keeping them balanced through a combination of personalized medicine, lifestyle changes, and emerging therapies can add years to your life—and life to your years. So, whether it's sipping green tea, lifting weights, or meditating, every little action contributes to the harmony of your longevity journey. Here's to make every note count!

CHAPTER 10 COGNITIVE HEALTH AND BRAIN LONGEVITY

Your brain, the command center of your body, is also the ultimate multitasker–juggling memories, emotions, logic, and creativity while ensuring you breathe and blink on time. But as we age, this intricate masterpiece requires extra care. Cognitive health is not just about avoiding decline; it's about optimizing your brain's performance for the long haul. Let's dive into the fascinating science and strategies for a sharp mind and a long life.

10.1. Preventing Cognitive Decline: A Deep Dive into Brain Longevity

As we age, our brains naturally undergo changes. Some of these changes are expected, like slower processing speed or occasional forgetfulness. But understanding the mechanisms behind cognitive aging can help us take proactive steps to maintain and even enhance brain health.

10.1.1. Mechanisms of Cognitive Aging

Several factors contribute to cognitive aging, but three main culprits often take center stage:

- Neuroinflammation: Chronic, low-grade inflammation in the brain can gradually damage neurons, much like rust corroding metal. Over time, this inflammation can impair memory and decision-making. Think of neuroinflammation as an uninvited guest overstaying their welcome.

- Oxidative Stress: This occurs when there's an imbalance between free radicals (unstable molecules) and antioxidants (your body's defense system). Free radicals cause damage at the cellular level, leading to accelerated brain aging. Antioxidants act like your brain's cleanup crew, neutralizing these troublemakers.
- Neurodegeneration: The gradual loss of neurons—the brain's building blocks—can lead to conditions like Alzheimer's and Parkinson's disease. Think of it as your brain's workforce shrinking over time.

How to Fight Back:

- Diet: Incorporate foods high in antioxidants, such as blueberries, spinach, and green tea. These foods help neutralize free radicals and protect your brain.
- Anti-inflammatory Choices: Add turmeric to your meals; its active compound, curcumin, is a powerful anti-inflammatory agent. Pair it with black pepper to enhance absorption.
- Support Your Cells: Supplements like CoQ10 and magnesium support mitochondrial function, which keeps your brain cells energized.

10.1.2. Nutrients for Brain Health

Your brain thrives on specific nutrients. Feeding it properly is like fueling a high-performance car—the better the fuel, the better the performance.

- Omega-3 Fatty Acids: Found in fatty fish (like salmon and mackerel) and flaxseeds, these healthy fats reduce inflammation and improve communication between brain cells. They're essential for maintaining the structure of your brain's cell membranes.

- B-Vitamins: Particularly B6, B9 (folate), and B12, these vitamins help produce neurotransmitters, the brain's chemical messengers. They also reduce homocysteine levels, a compound linked to cognitive decline.
- Polyphenols and Antioxidants: Found in dark berries, coffee, and cacao, these compounds combat oxidative stress and may even slow the progression of cognitive aging.

Easy Tip: Snack on walnuts and dark chocolate—delicious, brain-boosting powerhouses.

10.1.3. Physical Activity and Cognitive Function

Exercise is not just for your muscles; it's a workout for your brain, too. Regular physical activity boosts blood flow, delivering oxygen and nutrients to your brain, and promotes the production of beneficial proteins.

- Neurogenesis: Exercise encourages the growth of new neurons, a process that is critical for learning and memory. It's like planting new seeds in your mental garden.
- BDNF (Brain-Derived Neurotrophic Factor): Often referred to as Miracle-Gro for your brain, BDNF helps neurons grow, connect, and thrive. Activities like brisk walking, yoga, or even dancing can stimulate its production.

Pro Tip: Aim for at least 30 minutes of moderate exercise most days of the week. Even a quick walk can do wonders.

10.2. Neuroplasticity and Cognitive Resilience: Build a Better Brain

Enhancing Neuroplasticity

Neuroplasticity is your brain's ability to adapt, rewire, and learn new things, a feature that's active throughout your life. Think of it as your brain's version of remodeling and upgrading.

To enhance neuroplasticity:

- Learn a New Skill: Whether it's cooking a new recipe, playing an instrument, or taking up a new language, challenging your brain keeps it flexible.
- Puzzles and Games: Engage in activities like Sudoku, crossword puzzles, or chess. These are mental workouts that strengthen your cognitive abilities.
- Creativity Matters: Painting, writing, or crafting not only enhances neuroplasticity but also reduces stress, a win-win for your brain.

Cognitive Training

Cognitive training programs have grown in popularity for a reason: they work. Apps like Lumosity or Elevate provide targeted exercises to improve memory, attention, and problem-solving skills. Consistency is key, a little brain training every day goes a long way.

Social Interaction

Humans are social creatures, and staying connected is vital for brain health. Social interactions stimulate various areas of the brain, keeping it active and engaged. Whether it's joining a book club, attending a community event, or simply catching up with friends, meaningful connections can reduce the risk of cognitive decline.

10.3. Nootropics and Brain-Boosting Supplements: The Brain's Secret Weapons

Nootropics, also known as smart drugs or cognitive enhancers, are substances that boost brain performance. While some are natural, others are synthetically designed.

Natural Nootropics:

Bacopa Monnieri: An ancient herb known for improving memory and reducing anxiety.

Lion's Mane Mushroom: Stimulates the growth of nerve cells and supports brain regeneration.

Synthetic Nootropics:

Racetams: These compounds enhance memory and focus.

Modafinil: Often used to promote wakefulness and improve concentration.

Evidence-Based Brain Supplements

- Ginkgo Biloba: Known to improve blood circulation in the brain and enhance memory.
- Phosphatidylserine: A phospholipid that maintains cell membrane health.
- Acetyl-L-Carnitine: Helps in energy production within brain cells, improving mental clarity and focus.

Tailor Your Stack: Customize your nootropics based on your needs; for example, choose Lion's Mane for neurogenesis or L-theanine for stress relief.

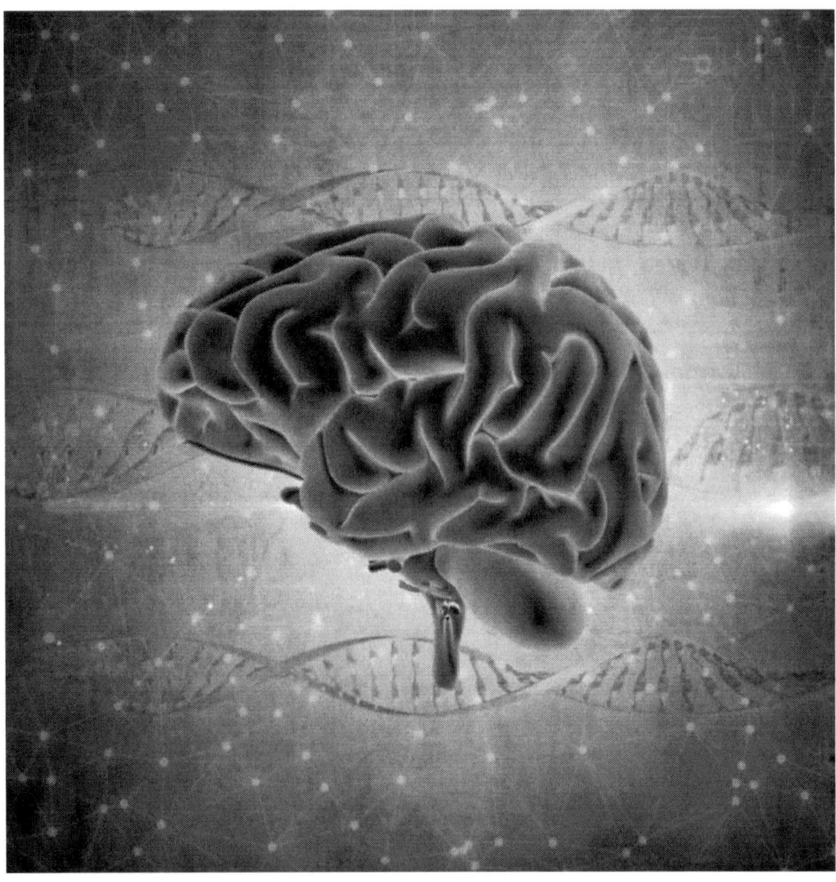

10.4. Mental Health and Longevity: The Mind-Body Connection

Mental health and physical health are inseparable. Chronic stress, depression, and anxiety can increase inflammation and oxidative stress, accelerating aging and cognitive decline. Addressing mental health is not just about feeling good, it's about living longer.

Integrative Approaches to Mental Health

- Nutrition: A Mediterranean diet rich in fruits, vegetables, whole grains, and healthy fats supports emotional well-being.
- Exercise: Regular physical activity releases endorphins, which are natural mood lifters.
- Mind-Body Practices: Practices like meditation, deep breathing, and yoga activate the parasympathetic nervous system, reducing stress and promoting relaxation.

Purpose and Meaning

Having a sense of purpose is like rocket fuel for your brain. Studies show that people with a clear sense of purpose have better cognitive health and live longer. Whether it's through volunteering, mentoring, or pursuing a hobby, finding your "why" is key to overall health.

10.5. The Intelligence Hormones

Hormones are not just about metabolism or growth; they're vital for brain function and cognition. Here are five key intelligence hormones and how they influence your brain:

1. Dopamine: The Motivation Molecule

Dopamine is your brain's reward hormone. It drives motivation, focus, and feelings of accomplishment. High dopamine levels make you feel energized and sharp, while low levels can lead to lethargy and lack of focus.

How to Boost Dopamine:

- Celebrating small wins triggering the reward response.
- Exercise regularly; even a brisk walk can elevate dopamine levels.
- Eat dopamine-boosting foods like bananas, avocados, and almonds.
- Reduce sugar and high-fat junk foods that can disrupt dopamine balance.

2. Serotonin: The Mood Stabilizer

Serotonin promotes feelings of happiness and emotional balance. It also plays a role in learning and memory. Deficiency in serotonin can lead to depression and cognitive fog.

How to Boost Serotonin:

- Spend time in sunlight, natural light triggers serotonin production.
- Include tryptophan-rich foods like turkey, eggs, and nuts in your diet.
- Engage in activities that bring joy, like listening to music or practicing gratitude.

3. Oxytocin: The Bonding Hormone

Known as the "love hormone," oxytocin fosters social bonding and trust. It's essential for building strong relationships, which in turn enhances cognitive resilience.

How to Boost Oxytocin:

- Engage in meaningful social interactions and physical touch, like hugs.
- Practice kindness and empathy; helping others can increase oxytocin levels.
- Meditate or practice mindfulness to enhance feelings of connection.

4. BDNF: The Brain's Miracle-Gro

Brain-Derived Neurotrophic Factor (BDNF) is a protein often referred to as "fertilizer for the brain." It supports the growth and survival of neurons, enhancing learning, memory, and overall brain plasticity.

How to Boost BDNF:

- Exercise, particularly aerobic activities like running or cycling.
- Incorporate intermittent fasting; studies show it can increase BDNF levels.
- Eat omega-3-rich foods and avoid refined sugar, which can lower BDNF production.

5. Cortisol: The Stress Hormone

While cortisol is necessary in small amounts for energy and alertness, chronic stress can lead to an overproduction of cortisol, which damages neurons and impairs memory.

How to Balance Cortisol:

- Practice stress management techniques like meditation and deep breathing.
- Prioritize sleep; aim for 7-9 hours of quality rest.
- Consume adaptogens like ashwagandha and rhodiola, which help regulate cortisol levels.

By optimizing these hormones, you create a brain-friendly environment that supports cognitive function and longevity. Balance is key: too much or too little of any hormone can throw your system off-kilter. Combine these strategies with a healthy lifestyle for a brain that thrives at every stage of life.

In summary, brain longevity is a blend of science and lifestyle. From nurturing neuroplasticity to embracing nootropics, the choices you make today can keep your brain youthful for decades. So, go ahead—pick up that Sudoku, lace up your sneakers, and maybe snack on some dark chocolate while you're at it. Your future self will thank you.

CHAPTER 11
CARDIOMETABOLIC VITALITY

Cardiometabolic health is the bedrock of a long and vibrant life. It's where the heart's rhythmic beats meet the metabolic orchestra that fuels our bodies. But this intricate system isn't self-sustaining; it requires conscious effort to thrive. Welcome to the fusion of functional medicine and cardiometabolic vitality. A journey into understanding, optimizing, and safeguarding the delicate balance that keeps us alive and thriving.

11.1. Understanding Cardiometabolic Health

Introduction to Cardiometabolic Health

Cardiometabolic health refers to the interwoven relationship between cardiovascular function and metabolic processes. Imagine your heart and metabolism as dance partners, perfectly synchronized, ensuring that oxygen, nutrients, and energy flow seamlessly through your body. This system regulates vital factors like blood pressure, cholesterol, blood sugar, and insulin sensitivity, and when it's in harmony, it's like a symphony. But if one instrument falters, the entire performance suffers.

Key Components: Cardiovascular and Metabolic Systems

The cardiovascular system, comprising the heart and blood vessels, works together with the metabolic system—a complex network that regulates how we process energy. Together, they influence everything from how we convert food into fuel to how efficiently blood delivers nutrients. Understanding this synergy is the first step toward achieving cardiometabolic vitality.

Obesity: A Major Risk Factor for Cardiometabolic Health

Obesity isn't just about extra weight, it's a powerful disruptor of cardiometabolic health, significantly increasing the risk of conditions like heart disease, hypertension, type 2 diabetes, and metabolic syndrome. Excess body fat, especially visceral fat around the abdomen, acts as an active endocrine organ, releasing inflammatory cytokines and disrupting hormonal balance. This chronic low-grade inflammation contributes to insulin resistance, arterial stiffness, and dyslipidemia, setting the stage for serious cardiovascular and metabolic complications.

One of the key mechanisms linking obesity to poor cardiometabolic health is insulin resistance. As fat accumulates, especially in muscle and liver cells, the body becomes less responsive to insulin, forcing the pancreas to work overtime to produce more. Over time, this leads to persistently high blood sugar levels and an increased risk of type 2 diabetes. Simultaneously, excess adipose tissue raises triglycerides, lowers protective HDL cholesterol, and promotes plaque buildup in arteries, significantly increasing the likelihood of heart attacks and strokes.

Beyond the metabolic disruptions, obesity also puts a mechanical strain on the heart. The increased demand for oxygen and nutrients forces the heart to pump harder, leading to elevated blood pressure and, over time, left ventricular hypertrophy—an enlargement of the heart muscle that weakens its efficiency. Compounding this, obesity often coexists with poor lifestyle habits, including a sedentary lifestyle, ultra-processed diets, and disrupted sleep patterns, all of which further amplify cardiometabolic risks.

The good news? Even modest weight loss—just 5-10% of body weight—can lead to significant improvements in blood sugar control, cholesterol levels, and blood pressure. Strategies such as adopting a nutrient-dense diet, prioritizing movement, managing stress, and optimizing sleep can help break the cycle of metabolic dysfunction and restore balance. Understanding obesity as a driver of cardiometabolic disease underscores the need for proactive, sustainable interventions to prevent long-term complications and improve overall health.

11.2. The Significance of Cardiometabolic Health

Public Health Impact

Cardiometabolic diseases, such as heart disease, stroke, and type 2 diabetes, are among the leading causes of death globally. They're not just personal health issues; they're public health crises, straining healthcare systems and overshadowing other medical priorities. Preventing these conditions isn't just good for individuals; it's essential for society.

Health Consequences

Poor cardiometabolic health reduces both lifespan and quality of life. Conditions like hypertension, high cholesterol, and insulin resistance don't just cause diseases; they steal years of vitality and independence, leading to increased morbidity and premature mortality.

Economic Costs

Managing cardiometabolic conditions isn't cheap. From medication to hospitalizations to lost productivity, the financial toll on individuals and economies is staggering. Investing in prevention is a cost-effective way to reduce these burdens and foster healthier populations.

11.3. Key Cardiometabolic Conditions

Cardiovascular Diseases

The heart is the cornerstone of cardiometabolic health, and when it falters, the effects ripple throughout the body. From coronary artery disease to heart failure, cardiovascular diseases remain a leading cause of disability and death. Understanding their root causes—like arterial plaque buildup and high blood pressure—is critical to prevention.

Metabolic Disorders

Metabolic disorders like type 2 diabetes and metabolic syndrome are often intertwined with cardiovascular issues. Insulin resistance, a hallmark of these conditions, leads to elevated blood sugar levels, inflammation, and vascular damage. Left unchecked, these conditions exacerbate the risk of heart disease.

Overlapping Risk Factors

Obesity, sedentary lifestyles, poor dietary habits, and chronic stress are shared risk factors that fuel both cardiovascular and metabolic diseases. Addressing these lifestyle factors is the linchpin of effective prevention.

11.4. The Rise of Cardiometabolic Disease

Epidemiological Trends

Cardiometabolic diseases are rising at an alarming rate globally, driven by factors like urbanization, aging populations, and sedentary lifestyles. The modern diet, laden with processed foods and added sugars, compounds the problem, creating a perfect storm for metabolic dysfunction.

Contributing Factors

While genetics play a role, lifestyle factors like poor nutrition, lack of exercise, and chronic stress are the primary drivers of the cardiometabolic epidemic. Even socioeconomic factors—like limited access to healthy foods and healthcare—contribute significantly.

Societal Implications

The societal impact of these diseases extends far beyond individual health. Healthcare systems are stretched thin, and the economic burden, including lost productivity and increased healthcare costs—is staggering. Addressing this epidemic requires a multifaceted approach involving public policy, education, and personal accountability.

11.5. Importance of Prevention and Management

Preventive Strategies

Prevention is the most powerful tool we have. Lifestyle modifications like healthy eating, regular exercise, and early screenings for risk factors can dramatically reduce the incidence of cardiometabolic diseases.

Holistic Approach

Functional medicine emphasizes treating root causes rather than just symptoms. This holistic approach integrates diet, exercise, stress management, and even mindfulness to optimize cardiometabolic health.

Long-Term Health Outcomes

Preventive measures don't just add years to life—they add life to years. Optimizing cardiometabolic health enhances overall well-being, allowing individuals to age with vitality and independence.

11.6. Lifestyle Interventions for Cardiometabolic Health

Optimizing cardiometabolic health isn't just about one factor—it's a symphony of diet, movement, rest, stress resilience, and brain support. Each pillar plays a crucial role in regulating metabolism, reducing inflammation, and enhancing overall vitality.

Diet: Fueling Metabolic and Cognitive Health

A nutrient-dense diet lays the foundation for cardiometabolic wellness. Prioritize whole foods rich in fiber, healthy fats, and lean proteins while minimizing refined sugars, processed foods, and trans fats, which contribute to insulin resistance and inflammation. Omega-3 fatty acids from fatty fish, nuts, and seeds support heart and brain health, while polyphenol-rich foods like berries, dark chocolate, and green tea provide antioxidant protection. Magnesium threonate, a highly bioavailable form of magnesium, supports neuronal function, stress resilience, and cognitive clarity, making it a key player in metabolic and brain health.

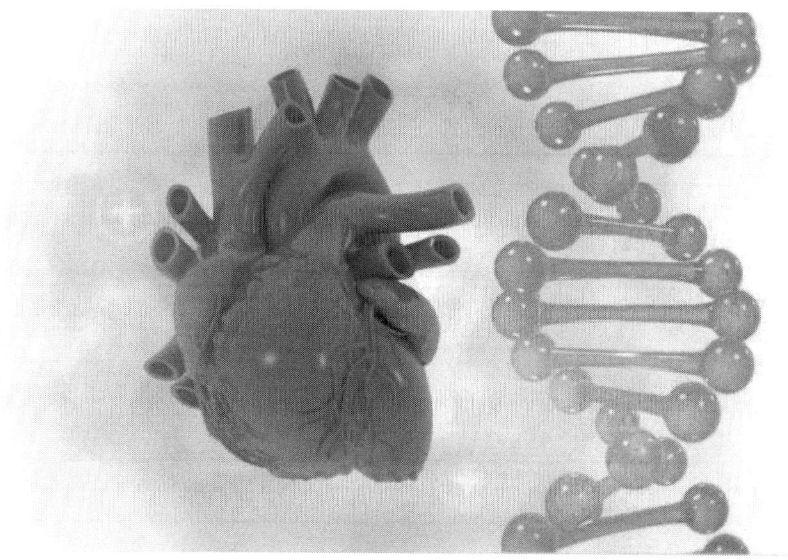

Exercise: A Metabolic Powerhouse

Physical activity is a cornerstone of cardiometabolic health. Aerobic exercise (walking, running, cycling) improves insulin sensitivity and cardiovascular function, while resistance training builds lean muscle, enhancing metabolic efficiency.

Movement also stimulates brain-derived neurotrophic factor (BDNF), which supports cognitive function, memory, and neuroplasticity.

Sleep: The Underestimated Metabolic Regulator

Poor sleep wreaks havoc on metabolic balance by disrupting hunger hormones (ghrelin and leptin), increasing cravings for high-calorie foods, and impairing glucose metabolism. Aim for 7-9 hours of high-quality sleep by prioritizing a dark, cool sleeping environment and maintaining a consistent bedtime routine. Phosphatidylserine, a phospholipid found in brain cell membranes, can help regulate cortisol levels, reduce stress-related sleep disturbances, and enhance cognitive function.

Stress Management: Keeping Cortisol in Check

Chronic stress drives up cortisol, which can lead to increased fat storage, insulin resistance, and cardiovascular strain. Managing stress is essential for metabolic balance. Mindfulness practices, meditation, yoga, deep breathing (such as somatic breathwork), and nature exposure are powerful tools to counteract the effects of chronic stress. Nutrients like magnesium threonate and phosphatidylserine help modulate the body's stress response, supporting both relaxation and brain function.

A holistic approach to cardiometabolic health requires not only optimizing diet and movement but also ensuring proper sleep, stress management, and brain support. By incorporating key nutrients like magnesium threonate and phosphatidylserine alongside lifestyle interventions, we can enhance metabolic function, protect cognitive health, and promote long-term well-being.

11.7. Nutritional Approaches for Cardiometabolic Health

Role of Nutrition

Nutrition is foundational for managing blood pressure, cholesterol, and blood sugar while reducing inflammation. A balanced diet rich in fiber, healthy fats, and plant-based proteins can prevent and even reverse many cardiometabolic conditions.

Interventions for Longevity

Calorie restriction and intermittent fasting stimulate cellular repair mechanisms like autophagy, enhancing longevity. Adopting diets that prioritize whole foods over processed options is a sustainable way to optimize health.

11.8. Integrative Therapies and Modalities

Holistic Frameworks

Integrating conventional medicine with lifestyle interventions and complementary therapies provides a comprehensive approach to cardiometabolic health. Practices like acupuncture, massage, and mindfulness complement traditional treatments.

Evidence-Based Modalities

From dietary changes to pharmacological interventions, evidence-based strategies like DASH (Dietary Approaches to Stop Hypertension) and tailored exercise programs are proven to improve cardiometabolic markers.

11.9. Future Directions and Emerging Research

Cutting-Edge Developments

Personalized medicine, integrating genomic data and advanced diagnostics, is paving the way for tailored interventions in cardiometabolic health. Imagine a future where wearable devices provide real-time insights into your metabolic health.

Promising Interventions

Emerging technologies like implantable devices for continuous glucose monitoring and targeted drug delivery are game changers. They offer precision in managing and preventing diseases.

Future Implications

A shift toward proactive, patient-centered healthcare will revolutionize cardiometabolic health, reducing disease prevalence and healthcare costs while improving quality of life.

11.10. Conclusion and Action Plan

Key Insights and Recommendations

Proactive measures, personalized approaches, and lifestyle changes are the pillars of cardiometabolic vitality. Prevention is not just a choice; it's a necessity.

Personalized Action Plan

Developing a personalized action plan involves assessing your current health, setting specific goals, and implementing lifestyle changes. Regular monitoring with biomarkers and health assessments ensures you stay on track.

In the end, cardiometabolic health isn't just about living longer, it's about living better. Start today, because every choice you make contributes to a healthier, more vibrant future.

CHAPTER 12
TOP LONGEVITY FOODS

Eat Your Way to Extra Years

The pursuit of a long and healthy life is no longer just the stuff of myths and fairy tales. Science has paved the way, and the roadmap is surprisingly delicious. One of the most critical factors influencing how long and how well we live is nutrition. What's on your plate doesn't just fill your belly—it holds the power to turn back the clock on aging, prevent chronic diseases, and keep your body humming like a well-oiled machine.

Functional medicine, a holistic approach to healthcare, places a spotlight on diet as the cornerstone of health and longevity. By focusing on nutrient-dense foods, we can not only extend our lifespan but also improve our quality of life. Ready to dive into the smorgasbord of life-enhancing eats? Let's take a closer look at the foods that can help you live longer, healthier, and better.

12.1. The Science Behind Longevity and Diet

Think of your body as a high-performance vehicle: it needs the right fuel to run smoothly and avoid breakdowns. Every bite you take influences your body's intricate biochemical processes, from cellular repair and regeneration to immune defense and energy production.

A nutrient-rich diet supports these processes, staving off inflammation, oxidative stress, and cellular aging that can lead to chronic diseases like heart disease, diabetes, and cancer. On the flip side, poor food choices can accelerate these processes, leaving you vulnerable to disease and premature aging. But there's good news: by making smart dietary choices, you can essentially "hack" your aging process.

Modern research highlights that nutrients play a pivotal role in modulating aging pathways like insulin signaling, oxidative stress reduction, and inflammatory response. By targeting these pathways, we can slow the hands of time and extend not only our lifespan but also our "healthspan"—the number of years we live free from disease.

12.1.1. Antioxidants: Your Cellular Bodyguards

Antioxidants are the first line of defense against oxidative stress, a major contributor to aging and chronic disease. Oxidative stress occurs when free radicals—unstable molecules that damage cells—outnumber antioxidants in your body. The result? Cellular chaos, premature aging, and increased disease risk.

Foods rich in antioxidants act like a cleanup crew, neutralizing free radicals before they wreak havoc. Fruits like blueberries, strawberries, and oranges are antioxidant powerhouses, boasting compounds like vitamin C, flavonoids, and anthocyanins. Vegetables like kale and spinach also pack a serious antioxidant punch, with compounds such as beta-carotene and lutein.

Notably, nuts and seeds like walnuts, almonds, and sunflower seeds provide vitamin E, a fat-soluble antioxidant that protects cell membranes. A diet rich in these foods can reduce inflammation, enhance skin elasticity, and even improve cognitive function.

12.1.2. Omega-3 Fatty Acids: Fats That Heal

Omega-3 fatty acids are essential fats that your body cannot produce on its own, making them a dietary must-have. These fats are known for their ability to reduce inflammation, improve heart health, and support brain function.

Fatty fishlike salmon, mackerel, and sardines are rich in EPA and DHA, two types of omega-3s that are especially beneficial. They lower triglyceride levels, reduce blood pressure, and enhance the elasticity of blood vessels, reducing the risk of cardiovascular disease. For those following a plant-based diet, chia seeds, flaxseeds, and walnuts are excellent sources of ALA, another type of omega-3.

Studies have shown that regular consumption of omega-3s can also delay the onset of neurodegenerative diseases like Alzheimer's by protecting brain cells and improving synaptic function.

Aim to include fatty fish at least twice a week or sprinkle seeds into your meals for an easy omega-3 boost.

12.1.3. Dietary Fiber: The Unsung Hero of Health

Fiber is a multitasking nutrient that works wonders for your digestive system, heart, and waistline. It comes in two forms: soluble and insoluble. Soluble fiber, found in foods like oats, beans, and apples, helps lower cholesterol and regulate blood sugar. Insoluble fiber, abundant in whole grains and vegetables, adds bulk to your stool and keeps your digestive system running smoothly.

But fiber's benefits don't stop there. It also feeds beneficial bacteria in your gut, creating a healthy microbiome that supports immunity, mood regulation, and even weight management. High-fiber diets have been linked to reduced risks of colorectal cancer, cardiovascular disease, and type 2 diabetes.

For an easy fiber boost, try starting your day with a bowl of oatmeal topped with fresh berries and a sprinkle of chia seeds.

12.1.4. Phytochemicals: Nature's Bioactive Compounds

Phytochemicals are naturally occurring compounds found in plants that offer an impressive range of health benefits. These bioactive compounds include flavonoids, carotenoids, and polyphenols, which act as antioxidants, anti-inflammatories, and even cancer fighters.

Tomatoes, for instance, are rich in lycopene, a carotenoid linked to reduced prostate cancer risk. Green tea contains catechins, polyphenols with potent antioxidants and anti-inflammatory effects. Cruciferous vegetables like broccoli and Brussels sprouts contain sulforaphane, a compound known for its cancer-fighting properties.

The best way to get your fill of phytochemicals? Eat a rainbow. Each color group offers a unique set of compounds that support different aspects of health.

12.2. Longevity All-Stars

Now that we've covered science, let's shine a spotlight on the foods that deserve a place on your plate every single day:

- Leafy Greens: Rich in vitamins, minerals, and antioxidants, these veggies are a cornerstone of any longevity-focused diet. They support bone health, eye health, and immune function. Pro tip: massage kale with olive oil and lemon juice to soften its texture and elevate its flavor.

- Berries: Packed with antioxidants and fiber, berries improve cognitive function, skin health, and digestion. Try adding them to salads or blending them into smoothies for a delicious, nutrient-packed treat.
- Nuts & Seeds: High in healthy fats, protein, and fiber, these snacks are a convenient way to support heart and brain health. Stick to one-ounce portions to keep calories in check.
- Fatty Fish: The omega-3s in fishlike salmon and sardines are game-changers for heart and brain health. If you're not a fish fan, consider a high-quality omega-3 supplement.
- Cruciferous Vegetables: Detoxifying and disease-fighting, these veggies are nutritional powerhouses. Steam, roast, or sauté them to keep their nutrients intact.
- Whole Grains: Foods like quinoa, brown rice, and oats provide sustained energy and support digestive health. They're also versatile enough to star in breakfast, lunch, or dinner.
- Legumes: Lentils, chickpeas, and black beans are high in protein and fiber, making them excellent for muscle repair and digestion. Bonus: they're budget-friendly!
- Fermented Foods: Probiotic-rich options like yogurt, kefir, sauerkraut, and kimchi improve gut health and enhance immunity. Add a spoonful of kimchi to your stir-fry or snack on yogurt topped with fruit and nuts.

12.3. The Art of Longevity: Meal Planning and Preparation

To reap the benefits of these foods, consistency is key. Meal prepping can save time and make it easier to stick to your goals. Cook large batches of whole grains and legumes, pre-cut your veggies, and stock up on nuts, seeds, and fermented foods.

Embrace seasonal eating to maximize freshness and nutrient content. Spring is perfect for leafy greens and berries, while fall calls for root vegetables and hearty grains. Rotate your meals to keep things interesting, and don't be afraid to experiment with new recipes.

Final Thoughts

A longevity-focused diet isn't just about living longer; it's about living better. By incorporating these nutrient-dense foods into your daily meals, you can support your body's natural defenses, boost your energy, and reduce your risk of chronic disease. Eating for longevity is both an art and a science—and the best part? It's delicious. So go ahead, savor every bite, and toast to a longer, healthier life!

CHAPTER 13
TOP LONGEVITY SUPPLEMENTS

Fueling the Fountain of Youth

Imagine living a long, vibrant life where your body thrives, your mind stays sharp, and aging feels less like a downhill race and more like a joyful journey. While no pill can turn back the clock entirely, science has uncovered a toolkit of supplements that, when paired with a nutrient-rich diet, can slow down the ticking hands of time. These supplements, backed by research, work to fortify your cells, reduce inflammation, and enhance the body's ability to ward off chronic diseases. Together, they form an arsenal against the effects of aging, giving you the energy and vitality to enjoy a long, fulfilling life.

But before diving into this treasure chest of longevity-boosters, let's address the cornerstone of health: your diet. A plate brimming with colorful vegetables, wholesome grains, healthy fats, and lean proteins is nature's gift to us. The Mediterranean diet and Okinawan diet are living proof that food is a potent medicine, with their emphasis on nutrient-dense, antioxidant-rich ingredients linked to some of the longest-living populations on Earth. Still, even the most perfect plate sometimes falls short, especially as aging alters our nutrient needs and absorption capacity. That's where supplements step in—not as replacements, but as reinforcements.

13.1. Magnesium: The Unsung Hero of Vitality

Magnesium is like the backstage crew of your body's health production—it may not take center stage, but without it, nothing would function as it should. This mineral is involved in over 300 enzymatic reactions, from supporting muscle function and bone strength to stabilizing mood and regulating blood sugar. As a natural relaxant, magnesium soothes the nervous system, reduces anxiety, and helps you sleep like a baby—key factors in maintaining long-term health.

Despite its importance, many adults fall short on magnesium due to depleted soils and processed diets. You can find this mineral in leafy greens, nuts, seeds, and whole grains, but supplementation is often necessary, particularly as stress and age deplete your reserves. Magnesium glycinate is a go-to for sleep and relaxation, while magnesium citrate can keep your digestion moving smoothly. Start with 200-400 mg daily and enjoy the peace this powerhouse brings to your cells and your mind.

13.2. NAD+: The Molecule of Youth

If aging had a kryptonite, NAD+ (nicotinamide adenine dinucleotide) might be it. This coenzyme fuels your mitochondria, enabling cells to produce the energy they need to function. NAD+ also plays a central role in DNA repair, maintaining the integrity of your genetic blueprint. Unfortunately, levels of NAD+ decline steeply with age, which contributes to reduced energy, slower repair mechanisms, and cellular aging.

Enter NAD+ boosters like nicotinamide riboside (NR) and nicotinamide mononucleotide (NMN). These supplements replenish NAD+ levels, revitalizing your

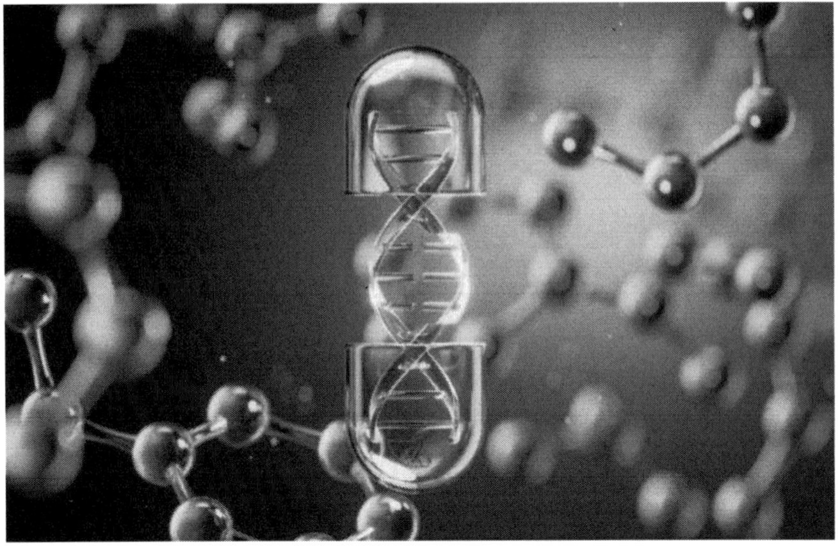

cells and extending their lifespan. Research has linked NAD+ restoration to improved energy, enhanced brain function, and even better metabolic health. Aim for 250-500 mg of NR or NMN daily to recharge your cells and bring youthful vigor back into your life.

13.3. Spermidine: Unlocking Cellular Renewal

Spermidine, a compound found in foods like wheat germ, soybeans, and aged cheese, has gained attention as a secret weapon for longevity. Its claim to fame lies in its ability to trigger autophagy—a cellular cleanup process that removes damaged components and rejuvenates cells. Autophagy declines as we age, leaving behind cellular debris that accelerates aging and increases disease risk.

By boosting autophagy, spermidine supports healthy aging at the cellular level, improving brain health, immune function, and even skin elasticity. While you can increase your intake of spermidine-rich foods, supplements offer a more concentrated dose to maximize its benefits. A typical dose of spermidine supplements ranges from 1-3 mg daily, making it an easy addition to your longevity toolkit.

13.4. C60: The Antioxidant Titan

Imagine a microscopic soccer ball kicking free radicals out of your system, this is C60, or Fullerene, a unique carbon molecule with extraordinary antioxidant properties. C60 neutralizes oxidative stress more effectively than most conventional antioxidants, shielding your cells from the wear and tear of aging.

Studies suggest that C60 can extend lifespan, improve energy levels, and even enhance physical performance. Its ability to reduce inflammation and promote mitochondrial health makes it a superstar for longevity. C60 is often infused into oils, like olive or avocado oil, for easier absorption. Start with a teaspoon daily and let this antioxidant powerhouse do the heavy lifting for your cells.

13.5. PQQ: Supercharging Your Mitochondria

If NAD+ powers your mitochondria, PQQ (pyrroloquinoline quinone) upgrades them. Known for its role in mitochondrial biogenesis—the creation of new mitochondria—PQQ boosts your cellular energy factories, keeping them running efficiently. This means more energy for you and less cellular aging.

PQQ also has neuroprotective benefits, supporting cognitive function and protecting your brain from the effects of aging. Found naturally in foods like kiwis, parsley, and green peppers, PQQ can also be taken as a supplement to supercharge your cells. A daily dose of 10-20 mg is typically recommended for those looking to boost their energy and brainpower.

13.6. D-Ribose: The Energy Spark

When your energy reserves feel depleted, D-ribose comes to the rescue. This naturally occurring sugar is a critical building block for ATP, the molecule that provides energy to every cell in your body. By replenishing ATP levels, D-ribose supports heart health, muscle recovery, and overall vitality.

D-ribose is particularly beneficial for individuals with chronic fatigue, fibromyalgia, or cardiovascular conditions, but anyone can benefit from its energy-boosting properties. You can find D-ribose in powder form, which mixes easily into water or smoothies. A typical daily dose is 5-10 grams, split into multiple servings to keep your energy steady throughout the day.

13.7. Adaptogens: Stress Resilience in a Bottle

Adaptogens, a group of herbs and botanicals, are like nature's way of saying, "Chill out; I've got this." These plants help your body adapt to stress, whether physical, emotional, or environmentally. Ashwagandha calms the mind and supports adrenal health. Rhodiola boosts energy and mental clarity. Holy basil reduces inflammation, and ginseng enhances physical endurance.

By balancing cortisol levels, adaptogens protect your body from the harmful effects of chronic stress, a major contributor to aging and disease. Incorporate adaptogens into your daily routine through teas, tinctures, or supplements. Dosages vary by herb but starting with 300-500 mg of ashwagandha or Rhodiola daily is a great way to begin building resilience.

13.8. Omega-3 Fatty Acids: The Peacekeepers of Inflammation

Picture this: your arteries are flowing smoothly, your heart is beating like a finely tuned drum, and your brain is firing on all cylinders. That's the magic of omega-3 fatty acids. These essential fats, found in fatty fishlike salmon and mackerel, and plant sources like flaxseed, act as the body's natural anti-inflammatory agents. EPA and DHA, the dynamic duo of omega-3s, not only reduce inflammation but also protect your heart, lower triglycerides, and sharpen your mind.

As you are aging, chronic inflammation sneaks in like an uninvited guest, wreaking havoc on your body. Omega-3s counteract this by calming the inflammatory response, paving the way for healthier arteries, clearer thinking, and a lower risk of neurodegenerative diseases. While a fillet of salmon twice a week is ideal, supplements can bridge the gap, offering a reliable source of these heart- and brain-loving fats.

For general maintenance, aim for 250-500 mg of EPA and DHA daily. If you're tackling specific health issues, like high triglycerides or rheumatoid arthritis, your doctor might suggest upping the dose to 2-4 grams per day.

13.9. Alpha-Lipoic Acid: The Cellular Dynamo

Deep within your cells, tiny engines called mitochondria churn out energy to keep you going. Alpha-lipoic acid (ALA) plays the role of both fuel and mechanic, boosting energy production while protecting your cells from oxidative damage. This dual-soluble antioxidant works in water and fat, reaching every nook and cranny of your body to neutralize free radicals.

Found in spinach, broccoli, and potatoes, ALA also excels at regenerating other antioxidants like vitamins C and E, creating a ripple effect of protection. Supplementing with ALA, especially as your natural levels decline with age, can sharpen your mental clarity, reduce fatigue, and support cellular longevity.

Most people benefit from 300-600 mg daily, though doses up to 1,200 mg may be recommended for conditions like diabetic neuropathy.

13.10. Vitamin D: Liquid Sunshine for Life

If sunlight feels like a warm hug from the universe, vitamin D is the gift left behind. Known as the "sunshine vitamin," it's critical for calcium absorption, bone strength, immune function, and even mood regulation. However, modern indoor lifestyles and geographical limitations often lead to widespread vitamin D deficiencies, especially in older adults.

Fatty fish, fortified foods, and supplements can help fill the gap when sunlight isn't enough. But vitamin D's benefits go far beyond bones. Research suggests it may reduce risks of heart disease, certain cancers, and autoimmune conditions. Simply put, this humble vitamin is a cornerstone of long-term health.

The sweet spot for most adults is 600-800 IU daily, though experts increasingly recommend 1,000-2,000 IU for optimal health. Check your levels regularly and aim to stay in the Goldilocks zone—not too low, not too high.

13.11. Coenzyme Q10: Your Cellular Charge

Imagine a team of electricians working tirelessly to keep your body powered. That's CoQ10, an enzyme vital for generating cellular energy. Found naturally in organ meats and fatty fish, CoQ10 keeps your mitochondria humming while shielding cells from oxidative stress.

As we age, CoQ10 production dwindles, leaving us more vulnerable to fatigue, heart issues, and even brain fog. For those on statin drugs, which deplete CoQ10 levels further, supplementation is a no-brainer. CoQ10 shines brightest in its role as an energy booster and heart protector, improving symptoms of heart failure and enhancing overall vitality.

For general health, start with 200 mg daily, and if you're targeting specific conditions, consult your doctor for higher doses. Remember, CoQ10 loves fat, so pair it with a meal for best results.

13.12. Curcumin: The Golden Healer

Bright, bold, and brimming with benefits, curcumin—the active compound in turmeric—is nature's anti-inflammatory powerhouse. Whether it's soothing arthritis symptoms or protecting brain cells from aging, curcumin's magic lies in its ability to inhibit inflammatory pathways and neutralize free radicals.

Yet there's a catch: curcumin's bioavailability is notoriously low. The solution? Supplements formulated with piperine or fats to improve absorption. Regular use of curcumin not only keeps inflammation at bay but also boosts brain-derived neurotrophic factor (BDNF), a molecule that supports memory and cognitive health.

For a daily dose of golden health, start with 500-1,000 mg of curcumin, ensuring your supplement includes a bio-enhancer like piperine.

13.13. Probiotics: The Gut's Secret Weapon

Your gut is more than a digestive machine—it's a bustling metropolis of microbes that influence everything from your immune system to your mental health. Probiotics, found in fermented foods like yogurt, kimchi, and kefir, help maintain harmony in this microbial city.

By bolstering your gut flora, probiotics reduce bloating, improve digestion, and even enhance immune resilience. They also show promise in slowing down aging by reducing chronic inflammation and supporting metabolic health.

Whether you enjoy them in your food or take them as supplements, aim for a variety of strains and a daily dose of 1-10 billion CFUs for general health.

13.14. Collagen: Building Blocks for Beauty and Strength

As we age, the body's collagen supply dwindles, leading to wrinkles, joint pain, and weakened bones. Supplementing with collagen peptides—derived from bovine, marine, or porcine sources—can replenish these reserves, restoring skin elasticity and fortifying bones and cartilage.

Regularly consuming 5-10 grams of collagen can reduce joint discomfort, improve skin hydration, and support overall structural integrity. For an added boost, pair collagen with vitamin C, which aids its synthesis.

13.15. Berberine: The Metabolic Multitasker

When it comes to managing blood sugar, Berberine is a heavyweight champion. This plant-derived compound activates AMPK, an enzyme that regulates energy production, reduces fat storage, and improves insulin sensitivity.

Whether you're tackling type 2 diabetes, high cholesterol, or metabolic syndrome, berberine delivers results rivaling some prescription medications while supporting cardiovascular and liver health. For best results, take 500 mg two to three times daily with meals.

13.16. Glutathione: The Master Antioxidant

Finally, we have glutathione, the unsung hero of longevity. This tri-amino acid compound is the body's ultimate detoxifier, neutralizing free radicals and aiding the liver in eliminating toxins. Found in foods like asparagus, avocado, and spinach, glutathione works overtime to keep cells young and functioning optimally.

For a health boost, consider supplements delivering 250-500 mg of glutathione or its precursor, NAC, daily. Combine with a diet rich in sulfur-containing foods like garlic and onions for maximum effect.

Your Longevity Toolkit

The road to a long, vibrant life is paved with small, consistent choices. By integrating these supplements into your daily routine, alongside a balanced diet, regular exercise, and stress management, you can fortify your body against the challenges of aging. Supplements aren't magic, but when chosen wisely and used thoughtfully, they're a powerful ally in your quest for health and longevity.

CHAPTER 14
ESSENTIAL LONGEVITY TOOLS

Building Your Arsenal for Vitality

Life is an adventure journey filled with twists, turns, and milestones that mark our growth and evolution. Along this path, the concept of longevity serves as a guiding light, illuminating the way toward a fuller, more vibrant existence. Longevity tools act as your trusty companions on this journey, not just extending the number of years you live, but enriching the quality of those years. These tools represent the art and science of aging gracefully, blending cutting-edge technology, ancient wisdom, and common sense into a toolkit designed for vitality, resilience, and purpose.

In the intricate tapestry of health and aging, longevity tools are the golden threads weaving vitality and rejuvenation into our lives. They range from dietary habits that nourish the body to mindful practices that nurture the soul. Each tool represents a unique avenue for sculpting a life brimming with energy and purpose. Aging doesn't have to be a slow decline—it can be a dance, where every step is purposeful and full of vitality. Ready to lace up those shoes? Let's dive into some of the most transformative tools in the longevity arsenal.

14.1. Infrared Sauna: Harnessing Heat for Longevity

Picture this: you step into an infrared sauna, and it's like a warm hug for your entire being. But this isn't just about relaxation, it's a gateway to enhanced well-being. Infrared saunas use gentle, penetrating heat to unlock a cascade of benefits that extend far beyond breaking a sweat.

At the top of the list is detoxification. Sweating isn't just about cooling down; it's your body's way of flushing out toxins and metabolic waste. Infrared saunas take this to the next level by stimulating sweat glands more deeply, helping to eliminate heavy metals and other harmful substances. This detox reduces oxidative stress and inflammation—two major culprits behind aging.

The benefits don't stop there. Infrared saunas also kickstart your circulation, delivering oxygen and nutrients to tissues while whisking away waste. This enhanced blood flow doesn't just rejuvenate your skin (hello, post-sauna glow) but also supports cardiovascular health and speeds up tissue repair. Add to this the production of heat shock proteins—your body's cellular repair crew—and you've got a recipe for resilience and renewal.

But let's not forget the golden rule of sauna use: hydrate, hydrate, hydrate! Infrared saunas work their magic through sweat, and replenishing lost fluids is essential for reaping their full benefits. Also, start slow, increasing your session length gradually to let your body acclimate. By following these simple steps, you'll be on your way to harnessing the healing power of heat.

14.2. Cold Plunge: Embracing the Chill

Cold plunges: the ultimate wake-up call for your body and mind. Plunging into icy water might sound like an extreme sport, but the benefits are worth the goosebumps. Beyond the initial shock lies a treasure trove of physiological and mental perks that make this practice a cornerstone of longevity.

Cold plunges are renowned for their ability to supercharge the immune system. The jolt of cold triggers a surge of adrenaline, priming your body to fend off pathogens with ninja-like efficiency. Regular exposure also increases white blood cell counts, bolstering your defenses against infections and diseases.

But the magic doesn't stop there. Cold plunges are a metabolism's best friend. The icy immersion activates brown fat specialized tissue that burns calories to generate heat. This metabolic boost doesn't just support weight management; it also improves nutrient delivery and cellular repair. And let's not forget the mental perks. The rush of endorphins post-plunge creates a natural 'high', enhancing mood, focus, and resilience.

Ready to take the plunge?

Start small. Ease your way in with shorter sessions and gradually increase your exposure. Listening to your body—there's a fine line between invigorating and overdoing it.

Pair your plunge with a warm-up routine and stay hydrated to maximize benefits safely.

The Controversy:

The cold plunge controversy dives into the heated debate over whether ice baths are a miracle hack for recovery, metabolism, and mental resilience—or just an overhyped trend with potential risks. Proponents swear by its ability to reduce inflammation, boost dopamine, and enhance resilience, while critics warn of cardiovascular strain, muscle recovery interference, and exaggerated benefits. The latest research suggests the truth lies somewhere in the middle: timing, individual health status, and duration matter. So, is it biohacking gold or just a chilling placebo? The jury's still out, but the ice keeps flowing.

14.3. Cryotherapy: The Cool Path to Longevity

Cryotherapy, or cold therapy, takes the chill of a cold plunge and turns it up... or rather, down. Exposing your body to sub-zero temperatures might sound intense, but it's a quick, effective way to reduce inflammation, speed recovery, and even improve mental clarity.

When you step into a cryotherapy chamber, your blood vessels constrict, redirecting blood to your core. Once you exit, blood flow surges back to your extremities, delivering oxygen and nutrients to your tissues. This process promotes healing, reduces swelling, and provides mental and physical refresh.

14.4. Light Therapy: Radiant Benefits

Light therapy is like sunshine in a bottle—or a lamp. It's a beacon of hope for regulating circadian rhythms, boosting mood, and even rejuvenating your skin. Whether it's natural sunlight or targeted artificial light, this tool is a game-changer in the longevity toolkit.

Circadian rhythms, your body's internal clock, dictate when you sleep, eat, and perform at your best. Light therapy helps synchronize these rhythms, ensuring you're in tune with the natural cycles of day and night. Morning light exposure boosts serotonin levels, giving you that feel-good vibe, while evening light encourages melatonin production for restful sleep.

And let's not forget the aesthetic perks. Light therapy, especially red and near-infrared wavelengths, promotes collagen production, reduces inflammation, and enhances skin tone. It's like hitting the reset button for your cells.

To integrate light therapy into your life, consistency is key. Start your mornings with bright light exposure to kickstart your day and wind down with softer, warmer light in the evening. Whether it's a walk in the sunshine or a session with a lightbox, let the light work its magic.

14.5. Hyperbaric Chamber: Diving into the Depths

Imagine a spa day for your cells, that's what hyperbaric oxygen therapy offers. By enveloping you in a pressurized environment, hyperbaric chambers flood your body with oxygen, fueling cellular metabolism and repair.

This therapy accelerates wound healing, reduces inflammation, and boosts brain health. Enhanced oxygenation promotes neural repair, improving memory and cognitive functional boon for anyone seeking to combat age-related decline. It's also been shown to support recovery from conditions like traumatic brain injuries and strokes.

Safety first, though. Hyperbaric therapy isn't for everyone, especially those with specific health conditions. Always consult a healthcare professional to ensure this tool fits seamlessly into your longevity plan.

14.6. Flotation Therapy: Weightless Wellness

Ever wish you could float away from life's stress? Flotation therapy makes it possible. Suspended in warm, salty water, you experience a sensory-deprived state that melts away tension and promotes profound relaxation.

By reducing stress hormones and promoting endorphin release, flotation therapy supports mental and physical recovery. It's a reset button for your nervous system, helping you face life's challenges with renewed clarity and calm.

14.7. Pulsed Electromagnetic Field (PEMF): Magnetic Healing

PEMF therapy might sound like science fiction, but it's grounded in solid science. By delivering electromagnetic pulses to your body, this tool stimulates cellular repair, reduces pain, and promotes overall wellness.

Think of it as recharging your body's batteries. PEMF boosts ATP production (your cells' energy currency), improves circulation, and reduces inflammation. However, not all PEMF devices are created equally. Analog PEMF, which generates smoother and more natural electromagnetic waves, is far superior to digital PEMF. Analog systems align more closely with the body's natural frequencies, offering deeper cellular benefits and fewer potential side effects. By contrast, digital PEMF devices can sometimes produce harsh, abrupt pulses that may not be as effective for long-term healing.

Whether you're recovering from an injury or seeking to enhance overall wellness, analog PEMF offers a powerful ally in the quest for longevity. Be sure to select a device that meets your needs and consult with a healthcare provider for optimal use.

14.8. Molecular Hydrogen Inhalation: Breathing Vitality

Molecular hydrogen inhalation is a rising star in the world of longevity tools, offering profound antioxidant and anti-inflammatory benefits. By delivering molecular hydrogen directly to your body through inhalation, this therapy targets oxidative stress—a major contributor to aging and chronic diseases.

When inhaled, molecular hydrogen neutralizes harmful free radicals, reducing cellular damage and supporting overall health. It has been shown to improve energy levels, cognitive function, and even exercise recovery. Best of all, it's a non-invasive, relaxing practice that integrates easily into daily routines.

14.9. Whole Body Photobiomodulation: Full-Spectrum Healing

Whole-body photobiomodulation is like giving every cell in your body a boost of sunlight without the UV damage. Using red and near-infrared light, this therapy penetrates deep into tissues to stimulate cellular energy production, reduce inflammation, and enhance repair mechanisms.

This therapy is particularly beneficial for improving circulation, boosting collagen production, and supporting mitochondrial health—all critical components of longevity. Regular sessions can enhance athletic performance, accelerate recovery, and even improve skin health, making it a versatile addition to any wellness regimen.

14.10. Synergizing Longevity Tools with Functional Medicine

Functional medicine personalizes health like a bespoke suit. By combining comprehensive assessments with targeted longevity tools, practitioners create a roadmap tailored to your unique needs. From optimizing detox pathways with infrared saunas to improving mental clarity with light therapy, the synergy between these tools and functional medicine is transformative.

Building Your Longevity Arsenal

Longevity isn't about finding the fountain of youth—it's about creating one within. By integrating peptides with tools like saunas, cold plunges, and light therapy with functional medicine's personalized approach, you can craft a wellness strategy that supports a vibrant, resilient life. Small, consistent steps today pave the way for a healthier tomorrow. So, what are you waiting for? Your journey to vitality starts now.

CHAPTER 15
FUNCTIONAL MEDICINE TESTING

Healthspangevity™ and Functional Medicine Testing

Imagine you're handed a map, but it's not for an exotic travel destination; it's the roadmap of *you*. It details the winding paths of your genes, the mountains and valleys of your hormones, and the bustling cityscape of your gut microbiome. Functional medicine testing is the GPS for navigating your healthspangevity™ journey—maximizing both your healthspan (the years you live well) and your lifespan (the years you live, period). By uncovering the mysteries of your unique biology, you can tailor strategies to unlock vitality, prevent disease, and age like fine wine (or at least not like a forgotten loaf of bread).

In this chapter, we'll delve into the fascinating world of functional medicine testing, explore the tests that matter most for healthspangevity™, and, most importantly, discover how to translate data into action. Get ready to geek out on health science while sprinkling a dash of wit and wisdom into the mix.

15.1. The Role of Functional Medicine Testing in Healthspangevity™

Why Testing Matters

Conventional medicine often waits for symptoms to sound the alarm before intervening. Functional medicine, on the other hand, gets proactive, digging deep into the root causes of health issues before they manifest. Think of it as fixing a squeaky wheel before it falls off the wagon entirely. Functional medicine testing provides insights that standard labs often miss: genetic predispositions, nutritional imbalances, hormonal hiccups, and more. This approach ensures you're not just putting out fires, you're fireproofing your health.

Personalized Health Insights

Let's face it: there's no such thing as one-size-fits-all health advice. While your neighbor thrives on keto, you might crash and burn. Functional medicine testing offers a backstage pass to your biochemistry, revealing how your body operates and what it craves. Personalized insights help you craft a game plan tailored to *you*, whether that means tweaking your diet, fine-tuning supplements, or doubling down on sleep hygiene.

Tracking Progress and Adjusting Strategies

Health isn't static. It's more like a playlist that evolves over time. Functional medicine testing is your Spotify Wrapped for health, showing what's working and where you're off-key. Regular retesting ensures you stay on track, allowing for course corrections as your body's needs shift with age, lifestyle, and external factors.

15.2. Key Functional Medicine Tests for Healthspangevity™

15.2.1. Comprehensive Blood Panels

- Inflammation Markers: Think of inflammation as your body's smoke alarm. Tests like High Sensitive C-reactive protein (HS-CRP) and erythrocyte sedimentation rate (ESR) measure chronic inflammation, which accelerates aging like an overzealous Instagram filter. Addressing inflammation helps maintain cellular efficiency, keeping you vibrant instead of prematurely worn out.

- Nutrient Deficiencies: Low on vitamin D or magnesium? That's like running a car on an empty tank. Nutrient panels assess levels of key players like vitamin B12, iron, and selenium. Correcting deficiencies fuels energy production, supports cognitive function, and keeps your immune system from staging a rebellion.
- Lipid Profile: Move over, basic cholesterol test. Advanced lipid profiles dive deeper, measuring LDL, HDL, triglycerides, and even particle size. This intel helps you tackle metabolic syndrome, heart disease, and other cardiovascular villains before they crash into your health party.

15.2.2. Hormonal Testing

- Thyroid Function: Your thyroid is the maestro of your metabolism. Testing TSH, free T3, free T4, and antibodies reveals whether it's in tune or hitting sour notes. A balanced thyroid keeps energy up, weight in check, and brain fog at bay.
- Sex Hormones: Hormones like estrogen, testosterone, and progesterone don't just influence mood and libido—they're architects of bone density, muscle mass, and even memory. Testing ensures these hormones are working in harmony, especially during transitions like menopause or andropause.
- Adrenal Function: Chronic stress is the villain in every health narrative. Cortisol testing (often through saliva) reveals how your adrenals are coping. If your cortisol

curve looks like a rollercoaster, it's time to address stress with targeted interventions.

15.2.3. Genetic Testing

- Genomic Analysis: Ever wonder why your friend can scarf down bread while you bloat just looking at a baguette? Genetic testing uncovers predispositions to conditions like Alzheimer's, cardiovascular disease, and metabolic dysfunction. Armed with this knowledge, you can tailor lifestyle and dietary choices to outsmart your genes.
- Methylation Pathways: Methylation sounds nerdy, but it's the process that powers DNA repair and detoxification. Testing for genes like MTHFR reveals whether your methylation game is strong or struggling, impacting everything from mood to cardiovascular health.

15.2.4. Gut Health Testing

- Comprehensive Stool Analysis: Your gut microbiome is like a bustling metropolis. This test identifies which bacteria are running the show—the good, the bad, and the downright ugly. Balancing your microbiome supports digestion, immunity, and even mental health.
- Food Sensitivity Testing: If you're perpetually bloated or fatigued, food sensitivities might be the culprits. Identifying and eliminating foods can reduce inflammation, improve gut health, and help you feel human again.
- Leaky Gut Testing: A leaky gut is like a castle with broken walls, letting invaders through. Testing the integrity of your gut lining can pinpoint issues

contributing to systemic inflammation and autoimmune conditions.

15.2.5. Advanced Cardiovascular Testing

- Coronary Artery Calcium Score: This imaging test measures calcification in coronary arteries—a predictive marker of heart disease risk. It's like peeking under the hood of your cardiovascular system to catch problems early.
- Advanced Lipid Testing: Beyond cholesterol, advanced tests like lipoprotein(a) and LDL particle number provide a nuanced view of heart health, helping you strategize more effectively.

15.2.6. Mitochondrial Function Testing

- Organic Acids Test (OAT): Your mitochondria are the power plants of your cells. The OAT evaluates energy production, detoxification pathways, and oxidative stress, giving insights into why you might feel perpetually drained.
- Nutrigenomics: Understanding how your genes interact with nutrients allows for precision in optimizing mitochondrial performance. It's like a cheat code for energy and longevity.

15.2.7. Telomere Length Testing

Telomeres are protective caps at the ends of chromosomes, shortening with each cell division. Their length serves as a key biomarker of aging and cellular health. Shorter telomeres have been linked to increased disease risk and accelerated aging.

15.2.8. Metabolic and Glycation Markers

Blood sugar regulation is vital for longevity. Poor glucose metabolism accelerates aging through glycation, damaging proteins and DNA.

Available Tests: HbA1c (Glycated Hemoglobin Test), Advanced Glycation End Products (AGEs) Test, Fasting Insulin and Glucose Panel.

15.2.9. Immune System & Senescent Cell Testing

The efficiency of the immune system declines with age, and the accumulation of senescent (zombie) cells promotes chronic inflammation.

Available Tests: Senescence-Associated Beta-Galactosidase (SA-β-Gal) Assay, CD4/CD8 Ratio Test, Natural Killer Cell Activity Test.

15.2.10. Bone Density & Skeletal Age Testing

Bone mineral density declines with age, increasing fracture risk and mobility issues.

Available Tests: Dual-Energy X-ray Absorptiometry (DEXA Scan), Trabecular Bone Score (TBS) Test, Osteocalcin and CTX Bone Resorption Markers.

15.2.11. Skin & Collagen Biomarkers

Collagen degradation contributes to skin aging, reduced elasticity, and decreased structural integrity.

Available Tests: Collagen Peptide Biomarker Testing, Skin Carotenoid Score (Antioxidant Measurement), Skin Elasticity and Hydration Analysis.

15.2.12. Biological Age Calculators (Multi-Marker Tests)

These tests combine multiple biomarkers to provide a comprehensive biological age assessment.

Available Tests: GlycanAge Biological Age Test, InsideTracker Biological Age Panel, Aging.AI Biological Age Prediction Tool.

15.3. Using Test Results to Create a Personalized Healthspangevity™ Plan

With the wealth of biological age testing now available, we can move beyond guesswork and into precision longevity optimization. By regularly monitoring these biomarkers, we gain valuable insights into how our body is aging and what steps we need to take to slow or even reverse age-related decline.

Personalized Interventions Based on Testing

The real power of biological age testing lies in the ability to take actionable steps based on the results. Depending on specific findings, interventions may include:

- Nutritional Adjustments: Enhancing anti-inflammatory, antioxidant-rich, and gut-supportive diets.

- Lifestyle Modifications: Improving sleep, reducing stress, and increasing physical activity.
- Targeted Supplementation: Using mitochondrial boosters, adaptogens, and hormone-supportive nutrients.
- Detoxification Strategies: Removing heavy metals, endocrine disruptors, and other toxins.

Interpreting Results

Getting test results is like receiving a treasure map—exciting, but potentially overwhelming. A skilled functional medicine practitioner is your guide, interpreting markers and creating a strategy tailored to your unique 'healthscape'. Whether it's replenishing magnesium or managing oxidative stress, each intervention is targeted and actionable.

Tailoring Interventions

The beauty of functional medicine testing is precision. Results might point to dietary tweaks (bye-bye, gluten), targeted supplements (hello, CoQ10), or lifestyle changes (yoga, anyone?). Each step is data-driven, ensuring your efforts pay off.

Monitoring and Adjusting

Health isn't set-it-and-forget-it. Retesting keeps you informed, ensuring you're making progress and catching new issues early. Think of it as recalibrating your GPS to avoid health detours.

Empowerment Through Knowledge

Knowledge is power, and functional medicine testing is the ultimate empowerment tool. By understanding your body's unique needs, you can take charge of your healthspangevity™ journey—living not just longer, but *better*.

Functional medicine testing is your backstage pass to optimal health. By embracing this proactive approach, you gain insights that allow you to tweak your health strategy with surgical precision. The result? A life filled with vitality, resilience, and the joy of knowing you're thriving at every stage. Here's to living well and long—because you deserve both.

The Future of Longevity and Health Optimization

The future of health isn't about simply living longer, it's about living better. By leveraging these state-of-the-art tests, we can craft personalized strategies that enhance vitality, prevent disease, and optimize performance at every stage of life. Biological aging is no longer a mystery; with the right tools, we have the power to slow it down, extend our healthspan, and redefine what it means to age well.

Your age doesn't have to define your health—your choices do. Start measuring, optimizing, and taking charge of your biological age today.

CHAPTER 16 THE FUTURE OF LONGEVITY

Where Science Fiction Meets Science Fact (and Maybe Some Zombie Cells)

The field of longevity is no longer the exclusive domain of sci-fi enthusiasts or dreamers hoping to outwit Father Time. With advancements that seem plucked from the pages of a futuristic novel, the journey toward healthspangevity™—maximizing both how long you live and how well you live—is entering a thrilling new era. In this chapter, we explore the cutting-edge research, innovations in personalized medicine, and ethical conundrums shaping the future of aging. It's a wild ride of hope, science, and some serious philosophical debates, so buckle up!

16.1. Cutting-Edge Research: Peering into the Aging Crystal Ball

16.1.1. Telomeres: The Protective Caps of Cellular Youth

Telomeres, the little end caps of chromosomes, are essentially the shoelace tips of your DNA. Just as frayed shoelaces spell doom for your sneakers, shortening telomeres spell trouble for your cells. Each time a cell divides, these caps get shorter, eventually signaling the cell to stop dividing or self-destruct. Enter the groundbreaking research into telomere maintenance, where scientists are uncovering ways to slow or even reverse this process.

Telomerase, an enzyme that rebuilds telomeres, is gaining attention as a potential anti-aging superstar. The hope? By boosting telomerase activity, we might preserve cellular health and extend not just our years but the quality of those years. Of course, the catch is ensuring this doesn't fuel the growth of pesky cancer cells. But hey, every good superhero has a complicated backstory, right?

16.1.2. Senescence and Senolytics: Dealing with Zombie Cells

If telomeres are the shoelace caps, senescent cells are the Halloween zombies of the cellular world. These "zombie cells" stop dividing but refuse to die, hanging around and spewing inflammatory compounds that wreak havoc on neighboring healthy cells.

Enter senolytics, a class of therapies designed to hunt down and eliminate these freeloaders. By clearing out these dysfunctional cells, researchers believe we can reduce inflammation, slow age-related decline, and maybe even give your mitochondria a little pep in their step. It's essentially a spring cleaning for your body, and let's be honest—who doesn't love the idea of a molecular Marie Kondo?

16.1.3. Mitochondria: The Power Plants of Youth

Mitochondria, often called the powerhouses of the cell, are the microscopic engines that keep your body running. But as you age, these engines can sputter, leading to reduced energy production and increased oxidative stress. Research into mitochondrial enhancement is tackling this issue head-on with therapies ranging from mitochondrial replacement to compounds like NAD+ and CoQ10.

Think of these innovations as upgrades to your body's energy grid, ensuring that you can run a marathon at 80—or at least dance through a wedding without collapsing into the cake.

16.2. Personalized Medicine: Your DNA as the Ultimate Cheat Code

16.2.1. Genomics: Decoding Your Blueprint

Your genetic code is like a set of IKEA instructions for your body—except way more complex, and you can't just toss it aside when it gets confusing. With advancements in genomics, we're learning how to read this manual better than ever. Imagine knowing which diseases you're predisposed to and tailoring your lifestyle and treatments to outsmart them. That's the promise of personalized genomics.

Even cooler, genomic testing reveals how your body metabolizes nutrients, processes toxins, and responds to exercise. Forget one-size-fits-all advice—this is health tailored to *you,* right down to how much broccoli you should eat.

16.2.2. Epigenetics: The Switchboard of Longevity

If your genes are the script, epigenetics is the director deciding which parts to emphasize or cut. These are the modifications that control whether certain genes are expressed or silenced, and the best part? You can influence them!

Lifestyle factors like diet, exercise, and even stress management can modify epigenetic marks, potentially slowing down the aging process. Think of it as your ability to rewrite your body's story—only this time, you're the editor-in-chief.

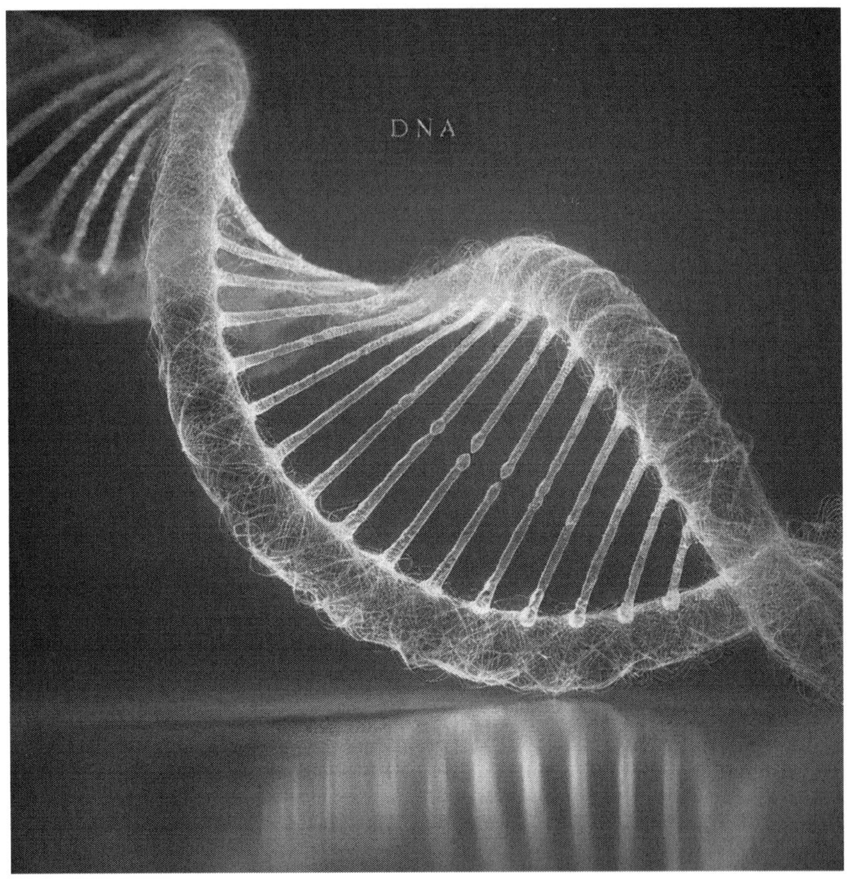

16.2.3. Predictive Medicine: Big Data and AI to the Rescue

Artificial intelligence (AI) and big data are transforming medicine in ways that feel borderline magical. Predictive algorithms can now forecast diseases long before symptoms appear, enabling early intervention. Want to know the likelihood of developing diabetes based on your grocery shopping habits? There's probably an algorithm for that.

The intersection of AI and longevity is also driving the development of highly personalized health plans, where your lifestyle, genetic data, and even wearable tech metrics are all combined to optimize your health like never before.

16.3. Ethical Considerations: Living Long and Living Right

16.3.1. Who Gets to Live Longer? The Equity Question

Let's address the elephant in the longevity lab: access. Life-extending therapies are exciting, but who gets them? Without careful thought, there's a risk of creating a world where the rich live long, vibrant lives while the less fortunate struggle with limited access. Ensuring equitable access isn't just a medical challenge; it's a societal one.

16.3.2. The Population Paradox: What Happens When Everyone Lives to 120?

Longer lifespans sound great, but what does that mean for population dynamics, resource allocation, and intergenerational relationships? Are we ready for a world where four generations are all job-hunting at the same time?

Balancing the promise of longevity with sustainable living is a puzzle we need to solve—not just for the planet but for our sanity during Thanksgiving dinner debates.

16.3.3. Quality vs. Quantity: The Aging Balancing Act

Would you rather live to 120 with your health intact or stumble painfully across the century mark? Longevity isn't just about adding years to your life; it's about adding life to your years. Making informed, ethical decisions about what we prioritize, quality or quantity—will shape how society embraces the science of aging.

16.4. Integrating Emerging Trends: Making the Future Work for You

Stay Curious: Longevity is a Moving Target

The field of longevity is evolving faster than your smartphone updates. Staying informed means following reputable sources, engaging in discussions, and, yes, questioning miracle cures that sound too good to be true.

Apply, Don't Overload

New discoveries are exciting, but they're only useful if applied thoughtfully. Start with one or two strategies that resonate with your goals and build from there. After all, no one wants to end up taking 47 supplements while neglecting the basics like sleep and hydration.

16.5. The Bottom Line

The future of longevity is as thrilling as it is complex. From zombie-cell-busting therapies to personalized genomics and ethical debates about resource allocation, we're living in a time where science is reshaping what it means to age. By staying curious, informed, and proactive, you're not just extending your lifespan, you're pioneering the future of healthspangevity™. So, go ahead—embrace the science, but don't forget to live a little while you're at it.

CHAPTER 17
CRAFTING YOUR HEALTHSPANGEVITY™ PLAN

17.1 Assessing Your Current Healthspan: Taking Stock of You

Before you start overhauling your diet, experimenting with 'biohacks', or downing mystery supplements, take a beat. First, you need to know your starting point—your healthspan baseline. Think of this as the diagnostic test before you tinker with the engine.

17.1.1 Key Biomarkers of Aging: Peeking Under the Hood

Your biological age isn't just a number on a cake; it's written in the biomarkers coursing through your veins. Here's what to track:

- Inflammation Markers: Elevated levels of CRP or ESR? Your body might be quietly simmering with chronic inflammation—an aging accelerant.
- Hormone Levels: Check thyroid hormones, sex hormones, and cortisol to uncover imbalances impacting energy, metabolism, or mood.
- Metabolic Indicators: Fasting blood glucose, insulin, and HbA1c aren't just for diabetics, they reveal how well you're managing blood sugar and fending off metabolic syndrome.

Continuous Glucose Monitoring (CGM) provides real-time insights into blood sugar levels, empowering individuals to make informed dietary and lifestyle choices for optimal metabolic health

17.1.2 Functional Medicine Assessments: The Deep Dive

Move beyond basic labs with:

Comprehensive Blood Panels:

Detect nutrient deficiencies, lipid profiles, and markers of oxidative stress.

Genetic Testing:

Decode predispositions for conditions like Alzheimer's or cardiovascular disease and pinpoint how your body metabolizes nutrients or responds to exercise.

Lifestyle Analysis:

A deep look at your diet, stress levels, and sleep patterns to identify what's working—and what isn't.

Longevity labs, whether conducted annually or biannually, serve as a critical tool for proactively assessing and optimizing health. These comprehensive panels go beyond routine checkups, offering a deep dive into biomarkers that influence aging, inflammation, metabolic function, hormonal balance, and cellular health. By tracking trends over time, individuals can catch early signs of imbalance, adjust lifestyle interventions, and fine-tune personalized longevity strategies. Regular testing ensures that cutting-edge advancements in longevity science—such as molecular hydrogen, mitochondrial support, and epigenetic optimization—are integrated into a proactive health plan, empowering individuals to not just extend lifespan but enhance vitality and performance at every stage of life.

17.1.3 Setting Health Goals: Mapping Your Route

Goals shouldn't be vague platitudes like "get healthier." Instead, define concrete, measurable targets:

- Boost your VO2 max by 10%.
- Achieve optimal Vitamin D levels (50–70 ng/mL).
- Reduce your biological age by five years (yes, it's possible!).

17.2 Building a Support System: No Longevity Island

You might think healthspangevity™ is a solo game, but even superheroes have sidekicks. Building your longevity team makes the journey sustainable—and a lot more enjoyable.

17.2.1 The Role of Family and Friends

Whether it's a spouse reminding you to hydrate or a friend challenging you to a fitness goal, your inner circle can be a powerful motivator. Share your aspirations, recruit allies, and gently convert them into accountability partners.

17.2.2 Finding the Right Healthcare Team

Not all heroes wear capes; some wear white coats. Seek professionals who align with your goals:

- Functional Medicine Practitioners: Experts in root-cause analysis.

- Nutritionists: Tailor your eating habits to your unique needs.
- Wellness Coaches: Cheerleaders who keep you accountable.

17.2.3 Accountability and Community: Strength in Numbers

Join longevity circles, online forums, or biohacking communities where people "get it." Community support keeps you motivated and exposes you to new ideas, research, and practices.

17.3 Tracking Progress: Because What Gets Measured Gets Managed

You wouldn't start a cross-country road trip without checking your GPS every now and then. The same principle applies to your healthspangevity™ journey.

17.3.1 Regular Check-Ins

Schedule health reviews every quarter. Update your biomarker tracking and note trends, like improved blood sugar control or reduced inflammation.

17.3.2 Leveraging Technology

- Wearables: Monitor sleep quality, heart rate variability, and daily steps.
- Health Apps: Log meals, track exercise, and integration with blood sugar monitors.
- AI Platforms: Use predictive algorithms to catch health trends before they become problems.

17.3.3 Celebrating Milestones

Crushed your first 10K or optimized your lipid panel? Don't just shrug it off. Treat yourself—a spa day, a fancy dinner (anti-inflammatory, of course), or even a quirky celebratory Instagram post. Positive reinforcement works!

17.4 Adapting to Life Changes: When Life Throws Curveballs

Life happens. Maybe you've switched careers, had a baby, or hit a milestone birthday (hello, 50!). Your healthspangevity™ plan needs to be as fluid as you are.

17.4.1 Modifying Your Plan

What works at 30 might not work at 60. Hormonal shifts, energy levels, and even workout preferences change. Learn to:

- Pivot your exercise from HIIT sessions to yoga for stress relief.
- Adjust supplements as nutrient absorption wanes with age.
- Redesign your diet to match changing caloric and protein needs.

17.4.2 Lifelong Learning

Science marches on. Today's longevity hack might be tomorrow's outdated fad. Stay curious:

- Read the latest research.
- Attend conferences or watch TED Talks and Podcasts.

- Follow thought leaders in longevity on social media.

17.4.3 Building Resilience

Not every day will be smooth. Health setbacks can happen: a torn ACL, a flare-up of an autoimmune condition, or a prolonged stressful period. Bounce back with:

- Mental Strategies: Meditate, practice gratitude, or journal.
- Spirituality and Faith: Reading and Mediating on the bible.
- Physical Adjustments: Lighten the load—literally and figuratively—when your body demands rest.
- Support Systems: Lean on your team when times get tough.

17.5 Conclusion: The Continuous Journey of Healthspangevity™

17.5.1 Embracing the Functional Medicine Mindset

- Take a proactive, root-cause approach to health.
- View prevention as the best form of medicine.
- Infuse purpose into your healthy journey; it's not just about living longer but living well.

17.5.2 The Power of Curiosity and Community

Stay curious. Engage with like-minded communities. Share your story, inspire others, and soak up wisdom from those ahead of you on the path.

17.5.3 Act Today

Start small but start today. Whether it's booking your first functional medicine appointment, committing to a bedtime routine, or buying your first wearable, every step counts.

17.6. Resources to Supercharge Your Journey

Scan the QR code and visit our FREE Resources Webpage. Here you can find:

- ✓ Sample Meal Plans
- ✓ Get anti-inflammatory recipes with longevity in mind.
- ✓ Supplement Guide
- ✓ Decode dosages, safety, and quality markers for key supplements.
- ✓ Longevity Resources
- ✓ A curated list of books, websites, and courses to feed your brain.
- ✓ Scientific References and related articles

With this chapter's comprehensive framework, you're equipped to craft a healthspangevity™ plan tailored to your unique needs. Remember, this isn't just about adding years to your life; it's about adding vibrant, meaningful life to your years.

"Make positive, conscious choices daily."

Drs. Oseni.

REFERENCES

In alphabetical order:

Abbott RD, White LR, Ross GW, et al. Walking and dementia in physically capable elderly men. JAMA. 2004;292(12):1447-1453. doi: 10.1001/jama.292.12.1447. PMID: 15383516.

Adams SH. Emerging perspectives on essential amino acid metabolism in obesity and the insulin-resistant state. Adv Nutr. 2011;2(6):445-456. doi: 10.3945/an.111.001297. PMID: 22211198; PMCID: PMC3262640.

Akbaraly TN, Brunner EJ, Ferrie JE, et al. Dietary pattern and depressive symptoms in middle age. Br J Psychiatry. 2009;195(5):408-413. doi: 10.1192/bjp.bp.108.058925. PMID: 19880930.

Alencar RR, Cobas RA, Gomes MB. Dyslipidemia in type 1 diabetes: a marker of cardiovascular disease. Diabetol Metab Syndr. 2012;4(1):23. doi: 10.1186/1758-5996-4-23. PMID: 22546088; PMCID: PMC3434027.

Ali T, Chugh D, Ekavali. Herbal drugs and their effects on cognitive function. J Tradit Complement Med. 2015;5(2):100-107. doi: 10.1016/j.jtcme.2014.11.017. PMID: 25883519; PMCID: PMC4387693.

Alpert JS. The broadening field of preventive cardiology. Am J Med. 2020;133(7):e323-e324. doi: 10.1016/j.amjmed.2020.02.032. PMID: 32240776.

Ames BN. Micronutrient deficiencies and DNA damage. Mutation Research. 2001;475(1-2):7-20. doi: 10.1016/s0027-5107(01)00091-8. PMID: 11295150.

Anderson RM, Shanmuganayagam D, Weindruch R. Caloric restriction and aging: studies in mice and monkeys. Toxicologic Pathology. 2009;37(1):47-51. doi: 10.1177/0192623308329476. PMID: 19129529.

Appel LJ, Moore TJ, Obarzanek E, et al. A clinical trial of the effects of dietary patterns on blood pressure. N Engl J Med. 1997;336(16):1117-1124. doi: 10.1056/NEJM199704173361601. PMID: 9099655.

Arai Y, Takayama M, Gondo Y, et al. Inflammation, but not telomere length, predicts successful aging at extreme old age: a longitudinal study of semi-supercentenarians. EBioMedicine. 2015;2(10):1549-1558. doi: 10.1016/j.ebiom.2015.07.029. PMID: 26501160; PMCID: PMC4586713.

Balasubramanian P, Howell PR, Anderson RM. Aging and caloric restriction research: a biological perspective with translational potential. EBioMedicine. 2017;21:37-44. doi: 10.1016/j.ebiom.2017.06.015. PMID: 28666535; PMCID: PMC5544561.

Barja G. Mitochondrial free radicals and aging. Trends in Neurosciences. 2004;27(10):595-600. doi: 10.1016/j.tins.2004.07.005. PMID: 15374670.

Bauer J, Biolo G, Cederholm T, et al. Evidence-based recommendations for optimal dietary protein intake in older people. Clin Nutr. 2013;32(6):929-936. doi: 10.1016/j.clnu.2013.04.018. PMID: 23786752.

Baur JA, Pearson KJ, Price NL, et al. Resveratrol improves health and survival of mice on a high-calorie diet. Nature. 2006;444(7117):337-342. doi: 10.1038/nature05354. PMID: 17086191.

Belsky DW, Caspi A, Arseneault L, et al. Quantification of biological aging in young adults. Proc Natl Acad Sci U S A. 2015;112(30):E4104-E4110. doi: 10.1073/pnas.1506264112. PMID: 26150497; PMCID: PMC4522786.

Bennett DA, Yu L, De Jager PL. Epigenomics of Alzheimer's disease. Transl Res. 2018;204:38-53. doi: 10.1016/j.trsl.2018.09.003. PMID: 30267841; PMCID: PMC6246912.

Berr C, Richard MJ, Gey KF, Favier A, Bourdel-Marchasson I. Enzymatic antioxidants and cognitive decline in the epidemiology of vascular aging (EVA) study. Clin Chem Lab Med. 2009;47(3):263-268. doi: 10.1515/CCLM.2009.058. PMID: 19243213.

Beydoun MA, Fanelli-Kuczmarski MT, Beydoun HA, et al. Dietary factors are associated with cognitive function in middle-aged and older adults. Nutrients. 2015;7(12):10223-10248. doi: 10.3390/nu7125524. PMID: 26694440; PMCID: PMC4690089.

Beydoun MA, Beydoun HA, Wang Y. Obesity and central obesity as risk factors for incident dementia and its subtypes. Psychosom Med. 2008;70(3):346-353. doi: 10.1097/PSY.0b013e318165bee2. PMID: 18378874.

Blasco MA. Telomeres and human disease: ageing, cancer and beyond. Nat Rev Genet. 2005;6(8):611-622. doi: 10.1038/nrg1656. PMID: 16136653.

Blumenthal JA, Sherwood A, Gullette EC, et al. Exercise and weight loss reduce blood pressure in men and women with mild hypertension. Arch Intern Med. 2000;160(13):1947-1958. doi: 10.1001/archinte.160.13.1947. PMID: 10888968.

Boeing H, Bechthold A, Bub A, et al. Critical review: vegetables and fruit in the prevention of chronic diseases. Eur J Nutr. 2012;51(6):637-663. doi: 10.1007/s00394-012-0380-y. PMID: 22684631.

Bondi MW, Edmonds EC, Salmon DP. Alzheimer's disease: past, present, and future. J Int Neuropsychol Soc. 2017;23(9-10):818-831. doi: 10.1017/S135561771700709. PMID: 29065941.

Booth FW, Roberts CK, Laye MJ. Lack of exercise is a major cause of chronic diseases. Compr Physiol. 2012;2(2):1143-1211. doi: 10.1002/cphy.c110025. PMID: 23798298.

Brenner C, Boileau RM. Nucleotide excision repair genes and aging. Cell Mol Life Sci. 2020;77(7):1287-1300. doi: 10.1007/s00018-019-03326-3. PMID: 31925530.

Burdge GC, Lillycrop KA. Nutrition, epigenetics, and developmental plasticity: implications for understanding human disease. Annu Rev Nutr. 2010;30:315-339. doi: 10.1146/annurev.nutr.012809.104751. PMID: 20645850.

Bäckhed F, Ley RE, Sonnenburg JL, Peterson DA, Gordon JI. Host-bacterial mutualism in the human intestine. Science. 2005;307(5717):1915-1920. doi: 10.1126/science.1104816. PMID: 15790844.

Cahill L. Why sex matters for neuroscience. Nat Rev Neurosci. 2006;7(6):477-484. doi: 10.1038/nrn1909. PMID: 16688123.

Calder PC. Omega-3 fatty acids and inflammatory processes: from molecules to man. Biochem Soc Trans. 2017;45(5):1105-1115. doi: 10.1042/BST20160474. PMID: 28900017.

Campisi J. Cellular senescence: putting the paradoxes in perspective. Curr Opin Genet Dev. 2011;21(1):107-112. doi: 10.1016/j.gde.2010.10.005. PMID: 21123043.

Cano A, Fortuno A, Quesada A. Endocrine aging and cardiovascular disease. Menopause Int. 2010;16(1):29-33. doi: 10.1258/mi.2009.009047. PMID: 20331801.

Cao L, Chiao M. Molecular pathways: targeting cancer stem cells through reactive oxygen species. Clin Cancer Res. 2014;20(3):584-590. doi: 10.1158/1078-0432.CCR-13-0915. PMID: 23975884.

Caporaso JG, Lauber CL, Costello EK, et al. Moving pictures of the human microbiome. Genome Biol. 2011;12(5):R50. doi: 10.1186/gb-2011-12-5-r50. PMID: 21624126; PMCID: PMC3213154.

Carvalho C, Moreira PI. Oxidative stress: a major player in cerebrovascular alterations associated to neurodegenerative events. Front Physiol. 2018;9:806. doi: 10.3389/fphys.2018.00806. PMID: 29977276; PMCID: PMC6019295.

Castro JP, Jung T, Grune T, Siems W. 80 years of research on protein oxidation: from the identification of oxidized proteins to proteomic approaches in aging research. Arch Biochem Biophys. 2013;542:3-11. doi: 10.1016/j.abb.2013.01.021. PMID: 23380396.

Chan DC, McKenzie B, Colman G, Boushey CJ. Importance of vitamin D status and lifestyle factors on bone mineral density in older adults. J Nutr Health Aging. 2011;15(7):535-541. doi: 10.1007/s12603-011-0034-2. PMID: 21849637.

Chen R, Ovbiagele B, Feng W. Diabetes and stroke: epidemiology, pathophysiology, pharmaceuticals and outcomes. Am J Med Sci. 2016;351(4):380-386. doi: 10.1016/j.amjms.2016.01.011. PMID: 27079344; PMCID: PMC4932700.

Cheng HL, Medlow S, Steinbeck K. The health consequences of obesity in young adulthood. Curr Obes Rep. 2016;5(1):30-37. doi: 10.1007/s13679-016-0197-7. PMID: 26769885.

Chowdhury R, Stevens S, Gorman D, et al. Vitamin D and risk of cause specific death: systematic review and meta-analysis of observational cohort and randomised intervention studies. BMJ. 2014;348:g1903. doi: 10.1136/bmj.g1903. PMID: 24690623; PMCID: PMC3972410.

Chrousos GP. Stress and disorders of the stress system. Nat Rev Endocrinol. 2009;5(7):374-381. doi: 10.1038/nrendo.2009.106. PMID: 19488073.

Cohen HY, Miller C, Bitterman KJ, et al. Calorie restriction promotes mammalian cell survival by inducing the SIRT1 deacetylase. Science. 2004;305(5682):390-392. doi: 10.1126/science.1099196. PMID: 15205477.

Corder R, Douthwaite JA, Lees DM, et al. Endothelin-1 synthesis reduced by red wine polyphenols: implications for health. Nature. 2001;414(6866):863-864. doi: 10.1038/414863a. PMID: 11780056.

Corpas E, Harman SM, Blackman MR. Human growth hormone and human aging. Endocr Rev. 1993;14(1):20-39. doi: 10.1210/edrv-14-1-20. PMID: 8484342.

Costello LC, Franklin RB. Zinc is decreased in prostate cancer: an established relationship of prostate cancer! J Biol Inorg Chem. 2006;11(7):943-957. doi: 10.1007/s00775-006-0142-6. PMID: 16909251.

Cotman CW, Berchtold NC. Exercise: a behavioral intervention to enhance brain health and plasticity. Trends Neurosci. 2002;25(6):295-301. doi: 10.1016/s0166-2236(02)02143-4. PMID: 12086747.

Cunnane SC, Courchesne-Loyer A, Vandenberghe C, et al. Can ketones compensate for deteriorating brain glucose uptake during aging? Implications for the risk and treatment of Alzheimer's disease. Ann N Y Acad Sci. 2016;1367(1):12-20. doi: 10.1111/nyas.12999. PMID: 26766547.

Dahl WJ, Stewart ML. Position of the Academy of Nutrition and Dietetics: Health implications of dietary fiber. J Acad Nutr Diet. 2015;115(11):1861-1870. doi: 10.1016/j.jand.2015.09.003. PMID: 26514720.

Davies KJ. Adaptive homeostasis. Mol Aspects Med. 2016;49:1-7. doi: 10.1016/j.mam.2016.04.007. PMID: 27105828.

dr Cabo R, Mattson MP. Effects of intermittent fasting on health, aging, and disease. N Engl J Med. 2019;381(26):2541-2551. doi: 10.1056/NEJMra1905136. PMID: 31881139; PMCID: PMC7285169.

de la Monte SM, Wands JR. Alzheimer's disease is type 3 diabetes–evidence reviewed. J Diabetes Sci Technol. 2008;2(6):1101-1113. doi: 10.1177/193229680800200619. PMID: 19885293; PMCID: PMC2769828.

Després JP. Body fat distribution and risk of cardiovascular disease: an update. Circulation. 2012;126(10):1301-1313. doi: 10.1161/CIRCULATIONAHA.111.067264. PMID: 22949540.

Diekelmann S, Born J. The memory function of sleep. Nat Rev Neurosci. 2010;11(2):114-126. doi: 10.1038/nrn2762. PMID: 20046194.

Dinan TG, Cryan JF. The microbiome-gut-brain axis in health and disease. Gastroenterol Clin North Am. 2017;46(1):77-89. doi: 10.1016/j.gtc.2016.09.007. PMID: 28164855.

Eckel RH, Grundy SM, Zimmet PZ. The metabolic syndrome. Lancet. 2005;365(9468):1415-1428. doi: 10.1016/S0140-6736(05)66378-7. PMID: 15836891.

Elamin MH, Shinwari Z, Hendawi M. NAD+ and its precursors in aging and age-related diseases. GeroScience. 2021;43(3):1021-1034. doi: 10.1007/s11357-020-00300-2. PMID: 33043389.

Eliassen AH, Colditz GA, Rosner B, Willett WC, Hankinson SE. Adult weight change and risk of postmenopausal breast cancer. JAMA. 2006;296(2):193-201. doi: 10.1001/jama.296.2.193. PMID: 16835423.

Estruch R, Ros E, Salas-Salvadó J, et al. Primary prevention of cardiovascular disease with a Mediterranean diet. N Engl J Med. 2013;368(14):1279-1290. doi: 10.1056/NEJMoa1200303. PMID: 23432189.

Ferguson G, Sheldon J. Cardiovascular risk and cholesterol management: new perspectives. Br J Gen Pract. 2014;64(620):610-611. doi: 10.3399/bjgp14X682633. PMID: 25548311; PMCID: PMC4240093.

Fink HA, Ginsberg TB. Cardiovascular disease and osteoporosis: balancing treatment benefits and risks. J Gerontol A Biol Sci Med Sci. 2006;61(4):362-371. doi: 10.1093/gerona/61.4.362. PMID: 16611704.

Finkel T, Holbrook NJ. Oxidants, oxidative stress and the biology of ageing. Nature. 2000;408(6809):239-247. doi: 10.1038/35041687. PMID: 11089981.

Fontana L, Partridge L. Promoting health and longevity through diet: From model organisms to humans. Cell. 2015;161(1):106-118. doi: 10.1016/j.cell.2015.02.020. PMID: 25815990.

Franceschi C, Garagnani P, Parini P, Giuliani C, Santoro A. Inflammaging: a new immune–metabolic viewpoint for age-related diseases. Nat Rev Endocrinol. 2018;14(10):576-590. doi: 10.1038/s41574-018-0059-4. PMID: 30065258.

Franklin SS, Wong ND. Hypertension and cardiovascular disease: contributions of the Framingham Heart Study. Glob Heart. 2013;8(1):49-57. doi: 10.1016/j.gheart.2012.12.004. PMID: 25690304.

Freitas AA, de Magalhães JP. A review and appraisal of the DNA damage theory of ageing. Mutat Res. 2011;728(1-2):12-22. doi: 10.1016/j.mrfmmm.2011.07.010. PMID: 21840364.

Friedman J, Nunnari J. Mitochondrial form and function. Nature. 2014;505(7483):335-343. doi: 10.1038/nature12985. PMID: 24429632.

Gabay C, Kushner I. Acute-phase proteins and other systemic responses to inflammation. N Engl J Med. 1999;340(6):448-454. doi: 10.1056/NEJM199902113400607. PMID: 9971870.

Gardener H, Wright CB. Dietary factors and cognitive decline. Stroke. 2018;49(4):1015-1020. doi: 10.1161/STROKEAHA.117.018146. PMID: 29467176; PMCID: PMC5886177.

Godos J, Ferri R, Caraci F, et al. Adherence to the Mediterranean diet is associated with better sleep quality in Italian adults. Nutrients. 2019;11(5):976. doi: 10.3390/nu11050976. PMID: 31060394; PMCID: PMC6566614.

Gomez-Pinilla F. Brain foods: the effects of nutrients on brain function. Nat Rev Neurosci. 2008;9(7):568-578. doi: 10.1038/nrn2421. PMID: 18568016.

Grant WB. Using multicountry ecological and observational studies to determine dietary risk factors for Alzheimer's disease. J Am Coll Nutr. 2016;35(5):476-489. doi: 10.1080/07315724.2015.1080127. PMID: 26880680.

Guarente L. Sirtuins, aging, and medicine. N Engl J Med. 2011;364(23):2235-2244. doi: 10.1056/NEJMra1100831. PMID: 21651395.

Gustafson DR. Adiposity hormones and dementia. J Neurol Sci. 2010;299(1-2):30-34. doi: 10.1016/j.jns.2010.08.004. PMID: 20800929.

Halliwell B. Free radicals and antioxidants: updating a personal view. Nutr Rev. 2012;70(5):257-265. doi: 10.1111/j.1753-4887.2012.00476.x. PMID: 22537212.

Hanage WP. Microbiology: Microbiome science needs a healthy dose of scepticism. Nature. 2014;512(7514):247-248. doi: 10.1038/512247a. PMID: 25119291.

Harman D. Aging: a theory based on free radical and radiation chemistry. J Gerontol. 1956;11(3):298-300. doi: 10.1093/geronj/11.3.298. PMID: 13332224.

Haus JM, Carrithers JA, Trappe SW, Trappe TA. Collagen, cross-linking, and advanced glycation end products in aging human skeletal muscle. J Appl Physiol (1985). 2007;103(6):2068-2076. doi: 10.1152/japplphysiol.00670.2007. PMID: 17901242.

Hooshmand B, Solomon A, Kåreholt I, et al. Homocysteine and holotranscobalamin and the risk of Alzheimer disease: a longitudinal population-based study. Am J Clin Nutr. 2010;92(3):595-603. doi: 10.3945/ajcn.2010.29482. PMID: 20685947.

Horvath S. DNA methylation age of human tissues and cell types. Genome Biol. 2013;14(10):R115. doi: 10.1186/gb-2013-14-10-r115. PMID: 24138928; PMCID: PMC4015143.

Houston DK, Nicklas BJ, Ding J, et al. Dietary protein intake is associated with lean mass change in older, community-dwelling adults: the Health, Aging, and Body Composition (Health ABC) Study. Am J Clin Nutr. 2008;87(1):150-155. doi: 10.1093/ajcn/87.1.150. PMID: 18175749.

Hu FB, Willett WC. Optimal diets for prevention of coronary heart disease. JAMA. 2002;288(20):2569-2578. doi: 10.1001/jama.288.20.2569. PMID: 12444864.

Hyman M, Malek M. The UltraMind Solution: Fix Your Broken Brain by Healing Your Body First. Scribner; 2008.

Jeong SM, Choi S, Kim K, Kim SM, Lee G, Park SM. Effect of change in total cholesterol levels on cardiovascular disease among young adults. J Am Heart Assoc. 2018;7(12):e008819. doi: 10.1161/JAHA.118.008819. PMID: 29910199; PMCID: PMC6064851.

Kaeberlein M. The biology of aging: citizen scientists and their pets as a bridge between research on model organisms and human subjects. Vet Pathol. 2016;53(2):291-298. doi: 10.1177/0300985815591082. PMID: 26136707; PMCID: PMC4779180.

Kennedy BK, Berger SL, Brunet A, et al. Geroscience: linking aging to chronic disease. Cell. 2014;159(4):709-713. doi: 10.1016/j.cell.2014.10.039. PMID: 25417146; PMCID: PMC4252700.

Kiecolt-Glaser JK, McGuire L, Robles TF, Glaser R. Emotions, morbidity, and mortality: new perspectives from psychoneuroimmunology. Annu Rev Psychol. 2002;53:83-107. doi: 10.1146/annurev.psych.53.100901.135217. PMID: 11752482.

Kivipelto M, Ngandu T, Fratiglioni L, et al. Obesity and vascular risk factors at midlife and the risk of dementia and Alzheimer disease. Arch Neurol. 2005;62(10):1556-1560. doi: 10.1001/archneur.62.10.1556. PMID: 16216938.

Knight JA. Review: Free radicals, antioxidants, and the immune system. Ann Clin Lab Sci. 2000;30(2):145-158. PMID: 10800390.

Kong F, Lin K. Oxidative stress in cancer: a double-edged sword. Cancer Lett. 2010;289(2):174-185. doi: 10.1016/j.canlet.2009.08.016. PMID: 19716385.

Koyama A, O'Brien J, Weuve J, et al. The role of peripheral inflammatory markers in dementia and Alzheimer's disease: a meta-analysis. J Gerontol A Biol Sci Med Sci. 2013;68(4):433-440. doi: 10.1093/gerona/gls187. PMID: 22982688.

Lang PO, Samaras D, Samaras N, Aspinall R. How important is nutrition in adult neurogenesis? Clin Interv Aging. 2010;5:187-200. doi: 10.2147/CIA.S9956. PMID: 20628630; PMCID: PMC2907136.

Larsson SC, Orsini N, Wolk A. Vitamin B6 and risk of colorectal cancer: a meta-analysis of prospective studies. JAMA. 2010;303(11):1077-1083. doi: 10.1001/jama.2010.263. PMID: 20233823.

Le Couteur DG, Solon-Biet S, Cogger VC, Mitchell SJ, Senior A, de Cabo R, Simpson SJ. The impact of low-protein high-carbohydrate diets on aging and lifespan. Cell Mol Life Sci. 2016;73(6):1237-1252. doi: 10.1007/s00018-015-2112-4. PMID: 26538595.

Lichtenstein AH, Appel LJ, Brands M, et al. Diet and lifestyle recommendations revision 2006: a scientific statement from the AHA Nutrition Committee. Circulation. 2006;114(1):82-96. doi: 10.1161/CIRCULATIONAHA.106.176158. PMID: 16785338.

Longo VD, Panda S. Fasting, circadian rhythms, and time-restricted feeding in healthy lifespan. Cell Metab. 2016;23(6):1048-1059. doi: 10.1016/j.cmet.2016.06.001. PMID: 27304506; PMCID: PMC4924195.

Lourida I, Hannon E, Littlejohns TJ, et al. Association of lifestyle and genetic risk with incidence of dementia. JAMA. 2019;322(5):430-437. doi: 10.1001/jama.2019.9879. PMID: 31310296; PMCID: PMC6687260.

López-Otín C, Blasco MA, Partridge L, Serrano M, Kroemer G. The hallmarks of aging. Cell. 2013;153(6):1194-1217. doi: 10.1016/j.cell.2013.05.039. PMID: 23746838.

Maher P. The potential of flavonoids for the treatment of neurodegenerative diseases. Int J Mol Sci. 2019;20(12):3056. doi: 10.3390/ijms20123056. PMID: 31234355; PMCID: PMC6617157.

Mann N, Skeaff CM. Lipids and health: an update. Nutrients. 2016;8(5):312. doi: 10.3390/nu8050312. PMID: 27187435; PMCID: PMC4882689.

Mattson MP. Energy intake and exercise as determinants of brain health and vulnerability to injury and disease. Cell Metab. 2012;16(6):706-722. doi: 10.1016/j.cmet.2012.11.008. PMID: 23217265.

McEwen BS. Protective and damaging effects of stress mediators: central role of the brain. Dialogues Clin Neurosci. 2006;8(4):367-381. PMID: 17290796; PMCID: PMC3181832.

Miller AH, Raison CL. The role of inflammation in depression: from evolutionary imperative to modern treatment target. Nat Rev Immunol. 2016;16(1):22-34. doi: 10.1038/nri.2015.5. PMID: 26711676.

Monteiro CA, Moubarac JC, Cannon G, Ng SW, Popkin B. Ultra-processed products are becoming dominant in the global food system. Obes Rev. 2013;14(Suppl 2):21-28. doi: 10.1111/obr.12107. PMID: 24102801.

Mozaffarian D, Micha R, Wallace S. Effects on coronary heart disease of increasing polyunsaturated fat in place of saturated fat: a systematic review and meta-analysis of randomized controlled trials. PLoS Med. 2010;7(3):e1000252. doi: 10.1371/journal.pmed.1000252. PMID: 20351774; PMCID: PMC2843598.

Mozaffarian D, Hao T, Rimm EB, Willett WC, Hu FB. Changes in diet and lifestyle and long-term weight gain in women and men. N Engl J Med. 2011;364(25):2392-2404. doi: 10.1056/NEJMoa1014296. PMID: 21696306; PMCID: PMC3151731.

Nabavi SF, Daglia M, Braidy N, Nabavi SM. Natural products, micronutrients, and nutraceuticals for the prevention and treatment of Alzheimer's disease: recent evidence and future potential. Curr Top Med Chem. 2017;17(6):519-529. doi: 10.2174/1568026616666160727110622. PMID: 27476069.

Nasreddine ZS, Phillips NA, Bédirian V, et al. The Montreal Cognitive Assessment (MoCA): a brief screening tool for mild cognitive impairment. J Am Geriatr Soc. 2005;53(4):695-699. doi: 10.1111/j.1532-5415.2005.53221.x. PMID: 15817019.

Ngandu T, Lehtisalo J, Solomon A, et al. A 2-year multidomain intervention of diet, exercise, cognitive training, and vascular risk monitoring versus control to prevent cognitive decline in at-risk elderly people (FINGER): a randomised controlled trial. Lancet. 2015;385(9984):2255-2263. doi: 10.1016/S0140-6736(15)60461-5. PMID: 25771249.

Nho K, Saykin AJ. Alzheimer's disease biomarkers: imaging, genetics, and CSF studies. In: Galimberti D, Scarpini E, eds. Neurodegenerative Diseases: Integrative PPPM Approach as the Medicine of the Future. Springer; 2015:149-167.

Nicklas BJ, Brinkley TE, Houston DK, et al. Effects of caloric restriction on cardiometabolic risk factors in moderately obese older adults. J Gerontol A Biol Sci Med Sci. 2009;64(5):468-475. doi: 10.1093/gerona/glp001. PMID: 19228770; PMCID: PMC2669740.

Nixon RA. The role of autophagy in neurodegenerative disease. Nat Med. 2013;19(8):983-997. doi: 10.1038/nm.3232. PMID: 23921753; PMCID: PMC4154441.

Palmer BF, Clegg DJ. The sexual dimorphism of obesity. Mol Cell Endocrinol. 2015;402:113-119. doi: 10.1016/j.mce.2014.11.029. PMID: 25459133; PMCID: PMC4465278.

Patel C, Goyal R. Cardiovascular risk and obesity. J Cardiometab Syndr. 2006;1(2):91-94. doi: 10.1111/j.1559-4564.2006.05598.x. PMID: 17620421.

Perez VI, Buffenstein R, Masamsetti V, et al. Protein stability and resistance to oxidative stress are determinants of longevity in the longest-living rodent, the naked mole-rat. Proc Natl Acad Sci U S A. 2009;106(9):3059-3064. doi: 10.1073/pnas.0809620106. PMID: 19223593; PMCID: PMC2656140.

Ristow M, Zarse K. How increased oxidative stress promotes longevity and metabolic health: The concept of mitochondrial hormesis (mitohormesis). Exp Gerontol. 2010;45(6):410-418. doi: 10.1016/j.exger.2010.03.014. PMID: 20350594.

Rizza W, Veronese N, Fontana L. What are the roles of calorie restriction and diet quality in promoting healthy longevity? Ageing Res Rev. 2014;13:38-45. doi: 10.1016/j.arr.2014.01.003. PMID: 24462722; PMCID: PMC4038355.

Saeedi P, Petersohn I, Salpea P, et al. Global and regional diabetes prevalence estimates for 2019 and projections for 2030 and 2045. Diabetes Res Clin Pract. 2019;157:107843. doi: 10.1016/j.diabres.2019.107843. PMID: 31518657.

Sies H, Berndt C, Jones DP. Oxidative stress. Annu Rev Biochem. 2017;86:715-748. doi: 10.1146/annurev-biochem-061516-045037. PMID: 28441057.

Smith SM, Vale WW. The role of the hypothalamic-pituitary-adrenal axis in neuroendocrine responses to stress. Dialogues Clin Neurosci. 2006;8(4):383-395. PMID: 17290797; PMCID: PMC3181830.

Walker MP. The role of sleep in cognition and emotion. Ann N Y Acad Sci. 2009;1156:168-197. doi: 10.1111/j.1749-6632.2009.04416.x. PMID: 19338508.Walsh ME, Bhattacharya A, Liu Y, Van

Remmen H. The histone deacetylase inhibitor butyrate improves metabolism and reduces muscle atrophy during aging. Aging Cell. 2015;14(6):957-970. doi: 10.1111/acel.12394. PMID: 26414661; PMCID: PMC4726515.

Made in the USA
Columbia, SC
07 July 2025

40cacec8-dcf5-4ddc-8799-a937eca442d5R01